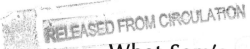

What Sam's
Are Sayin

D1240882

DATE

Sam's book *Keep Swinging!* puts forth the concept that we create our own lives. It doesn't just "happen" to us. To show how this takes place, Sam gives us concrete examples. The ones that grabbed me are:

A. That exercise can actually sustain and improve your mental condition.

B. Making it a habit to chip away at accomplishing your goals is the way to go.

C. The ability to take credit for your own successes can be like money in the bank.

D. It is clear that Sam benefited greatly from his mother's wisdom. I agree with Sam that one of the great pleasures in life comes from listening to the insights of older musicians, which can be viewed as beautiful shortcuts.

E. I find Sam's comparison between sports and music particularly valid because they both involve mental and physical skill. In addition both music and sports are "performance" occupations. Your job is to entertain.

> – Tom Olin, Saxophone and Clarinet Performer, Educator

You did it again! Once more you are giving us a wonderful perspective of your life philosophy. This book is full of good tips that will definitely inspire us. Reading your book is like taking your drum lesson; you always learn something!

> – Sebastien Amy, Author, Educator, Professional
> Percussion Player from France

Sam Ulano is a man with boundless energy. I have tremendous admiration for him.

> – Leonard Gaskin, Bassist, Educator

#23

If possible, your second book, *Keep Swinging!*, is even more out-standing than your first!

For me, it was a "Talking Document" that made for a quick and easy read, almost like you were with me in person. A virtual face-to-face discussion with a rare personality who has "been there and done that."

It taught me what song titles can mean:

"I've Got the World on a String"

"Que Sera, Sera"

"Love Is a Many Splendored Thing"

"When You Wish Upon a Star"

— and many, many more!

To sum up – your marvelous book is a "Literary Road Map for Happiness!!"

May the good Lord bless you in all that you do.

> – Arthur Scher, President, Scher Enterprises,

Once again, Sam offers a concise method of living which will optimize the vehicle called yourself.

> – Dr. Marianne Moy, Educational Specialist
> and University Professor.

Another remarkable achievement. Sam Ulano again challenges us to look within ourselves to find focus, motivation, and inspiration with his unique brand of philosophical genius. I love what YOU do too, Sam.

> – Stephen Korbel, Student, Musician, and
> Corporate Executive, Citigroup, Inc.

The ideas in this book are presented clearly, in a down-to-earth, wise, and witty manner.

> – Michele Zalkin, Educator

In *Keep Swinging!*, Sam Ulano shares with us the practical knowledge and wisdom of eighty-two years of life. Through his own process of self-exploration and self-reflection, he has provided us with viable methods to help cope with the many challenges that life presents. He reveals candid examples from his own life that can easily be applied to anyone facing challenges and obstacles in their life. Through his example, we are inspired to look within and discover our own unique potential.

This book is of benefit to persons of all ages who are seeking a more meaningful life. While reading it, I got the impression that Sam Ulano had become my own personal trainer, philosopher, psychologist, social worker, cheerleader, and coach. By "cutting to the chase," Sam Ulano has developed his own cognitive-behavioral approach to problem-solving and inner conflict resolution. This book will not only inspire you to find the "rhythm" in your life, but will give you the steps to dance to it.

– Michele Sarracco, MSW, CSW, Clinical Social
Worker/Psychotherapist

Sam's latest volume of philosophy once again proves he's got a lot more than rhythm going on. If we all have as fulfilling a life as Sam's when we're eighty-two, we'll be very fortunate indeed!

– Michael Greenberg, CSW, ACSW

Do you know "Mr. Rhythm" personally? When you finish reading this book, I am sure you will feel as I did. A friend, a good friend just gave me good advice.

Everyone deserves to be enlightened. Mr. Ulano's advice shines from the light. Consider yourself blessed as you hold this book, *Keep Swinging!*, in your hands. I do.

– Diana Nikkolas, Educator and Opera Singer

Sam Ulano has spent his entire life in music. Playing drums, teaching drums, and studying drums. Now at age eighty-two, he has shared his philosophy of life with us. This book promotes good life, well-being, and self-awareness. This is a must read for all!

– Dion Parson, Drummer and Educator

The most concise and to-the-point guide for productive and meaningful living through discipline, effort, and balance. Also, it is interspersed with reminders of all that is good and resonant that surrounds us everyday, which is there for the taking if you have eyes and a heart with the capabilities to absorb, as well as a capacity to be energized by its wonders.

– Ernie Ernst, President, Ernst Flow Industries

Enjoyed reading your book. A wonderful musician's view of life.

You have achieved musical success in your eighty-two-plus years in ways well beyond the dreams of most artists. Congratulations on assembling the keys to your accomplishments in your latest book. Anyone aspiring to a life dedicated to musicianship would learn a great deal by reading it.

May you continue to enjoy artistic success for many years to come.

– Fred Gretsch, President of Fred Gretsch Enterprises

This book has to be, "The Secret to Longevity in Life!" Motivation, Desire, Direction, and Faith have kept you young at eighty-two. Keep going in the same direction.

– Bill Rotella, Drummer, Teacher

Sam Ulano has written a wise and caring book packed with valuable ideas and information that have enriched my life.

– Al Warner, M.D., Pianist

Your philosophy in *Keep Swinging!* rings true. It's the common-sense stuff that is missing in households across this country. If parents model your philosophies you will see a new generation of kids. Their children will be physically and mentally healthy with respect of self and consequently of other. Not the me-me-me, video game-driven, self-centered, narcissistic kids we see around us. Thanks again for sharing your wisdom, and, as always, you remain my personal drumchiatrist.

– Eugene M. Kornhaber, M.D.

Sam nails it again. For those who know him, reading this book is like you are sitting next to the man. He practices every word that he preaches. Being Sam's student is like going to church. Hallelujah!

> – Scott Foley, Educator, Performer, Percussionist

I, too, feel that I have been blessed by the Good Lord with some talent [at eighty] and my brain is constantly working. Both Fred Gretsch and I agree that you offer great philosophy in your writing. We will highly recommend your book to all aspiring musicians.

> – Ernie Gadzos, Fred Gretsch Enterprises

The complicated made simple as only Sam could do.

> – Russ Moy, Performer, Educator, and Clinician

Thanks Sam for another inspirational book! Your commitment to sharing your outlook and philosophy of life with others is a blessing to all that read it. This book is unique because it discusses things that we all experience as people and frames those experiences in a very positive way. Thanks again Sam!

> – James Guarnieri, Performing Artist/Music Educator

This fine book by Sam Ulano contains really useful advice and grains of wisdom from a long and productive life. I've admired Sam's commonsense approach to life for a lengthy period of friendship. Good job, Sam!

> – Ed Shaughnessy, Professional Drummer,
> twenty-nine years on The Johnny Carson Show

I refer to the things I learned from Sam on a daily basis concerning life, music, business, and personal matters — twelve years after I finished studying with him. I value his knowledge immensely.

> – Vince Cherico, Ray Baretto's Band, Mury Recordings

In this complicated world in which we live, the most important aspects of life such as love, compassion, and honesty still remain timeless. Sam Ulano is a person who personifies the "art" of living. The gift of music, education, and unselfish giving are only some of the skills this man has mastered. His musical talents will never be forgotten by anyone who knows him. His ability to bring out the best in others in his teachings and writings is appreciated by the masses. The level of talent and knowledge that Sam possesses is truly conveyed through his written masterpieces. I am truly blessed to have experienced Sam's tutelage, along with his friendship, which has enabled me to become the musician and teacher I am today. I've been fortunate to experience his passion for educating and passing on his musical expertise to others. The highest respect and love go out to you, Sam!

Best wishes, congratulations, and KEEP LOVING LIFE!!!!

– John Sarracco, Drum Instructor and Performer

As in your music, Sam, so in your inspiring philosophy of life! Thank you for this outstanding offering, rich with your therapeutic voice and the accumulated wisdom of a life committed and dedicated to the spirit of music.

– John Diamond, M.D., DPM, FRANZCP, MRCPsych, FIAPM, DIBAK, Fellow and past President of the International Academy of Preventive Medicine, best-selling author of over 20 books, including *Your Body Doesn't Lie, Life Energy,* and *The Way of the Pulse: Drumming With Spirit*

Keep Swinging!

Approach Your Senior Years Without Skipping a Beat

Sam Ulano

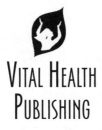

VITAL HEALTH
PUBLISHING

Keep Swinging! Approach Your Senior Years Without Skipping A Beat
Copyright 2005 by Sam Ulano

Cover photograph by Steven Korbel.

Published by: Vital Health Publishing
34 Mill Plain Road
Danbury, CT 06811
Website: www.vitalhealthbooks.com
E-mail: info@vitalhealthbooks.com

Printed in the United States of America
ISBN 1-890612-40-5

Table of Contents

Introduction   1
There Are Twenty-four Hours in a Day   3
Never Feel Sorry for Yourself   5
You Can't Spend More Than You Have   7
You Can Only Help Yourself. Each of Us Must Do It for
    Ourselves   9
There Is Always a Way To Do Something Better   11
As the Song Says, "Pick Yourself Up
    and Start All Over Again"   12
Have You Made Up Your Mind As to What You
    Love To Do?   14
Do You Change Your Mind Often?   16
Are You Flexible?   18
Do You Care for What You Do?   21
Does the Weather Affect Your Daily Life?   23
Do You Learn Something New Every Day?   24
Do You Go Back on What You Say You Will Do?   26
Make Rules for Yourself   28
Who Are You and Who Do You Want To Be?   30
What Is My Idea on How To Become an "Original"?   32
You Have To Work at Staying in Top Physical
    Shape Like an Athlete   34
There Aren't Any Shortcuts   36
I Believe You Must Get Your Inspiration from
    Within Yourself   38
Wishing Is Nice, but It Doesn't Work   40
Just a Reminder: Your Health Is Most Important   42
Have Patience in Whatever You Do   44
You Can't Discuss or Give an Opinion on a Subject About
    Which You Know Nothing   47
If You Are Going for an Interview,
    Make Sure You Are Totally Prepared   48

Listen and Learn   50
Think   52
You Can Exercise in Many Places   54
Don't Tell People What You Are Going To Do ... Do It!   56
Do You Have a Hobby   58
What Do You Think You Will Leave After You're Gone?   60
What Are Your Thoughts About Love   62
Are You a Gambler in Life?   64
Are You Certain That You Will Reach Your Goals?   67
The More I Think About It, the More I Realize
    the Importance of Our Legs   68
Do You Like Yourself?   70
Do You Believe There Is a Strong Power Watching
    Over You? Maybe Motivating You?   72
Are You Envious of Others?   74
Do You Study Yourself Day After Day?   76
Remember, the World Doesn't Owe You Anything   78
Who Motivates You?   80
Do You Believe in God?   82
Do You Know Where You Are Heading?   84
My Thoughts on Smoking and Drinking   86
How Do You Handle Holidays?   88
These Ideas Are All My Own   90
How I Changed My Life   92
If at First You Don't Succeed, Then You Only
    Have Yourself To Blame   94
Think Twice Before You Have Many Different Credit Cards   96
I Never Read Other Books About Philosophies of Life   98
Do You Take Life Too Seriously?   100
If You Succeed, All of the Credit Goes to You   102
Don't Borrow Money...You'll Be Sorry   104
If You Are in Charge, Be in Charge   106
How Do You Feel About Retiring   108
My Concepts About Retiring   110
You Know You're Old When You Retire   114
Only You Can Tell How You Feel While
    You're Getting Older   116

There Are Many Advantages To Being a Senior 118

I Have Lived in a Senior Center for the Past Sixteen Years 120

Don't Be Afraid of Growing Older 122

Have You Given Up on Your Desires? 124

Have You Become a "Couch Potato?" 126

Where Will You Spend Your Retirement Years? 128

As I Get Older, I Must Have Fun with My Life 130

Don't Live Only for Your Kids 132

You Have To Be a Bit Selfish 134

Study Yourself As You Get Older 136

Set Up a Purpose for Yourself 138

Take Care of Your Eyes and Ears 140

As You Get Older, You Will Experience the Same
    Things That All Seniors Do 142

I Am So Lucky To Be Alive and Still Doing
    What I Love To Do 143

Stay Busy and Involved 145

Are You Able To Handle Being Alone As You Grow Older? 146

If You Are Young, Have You Given Much
    Thought to How You Will Handle Growing Older? 148

Are You Keeping Active As You Are Getting Older? 150

Are You Going To Do All the Things You Wanted
    To Do As You Get Older? 152

How Will You Occupy Twenty-four Hours a Day? 153

Are You Expecting Your Kids To Take Care of You? 154

Keep Your Weight Under Strict Control 156

We Never Get Too Big To Stop Studying 158

You Don't Need Heavy Weights. 160

Never Stop 162

Why Say You're Going To Do Something
    and Then Never Do It? 164

Confidence and Conceit 166

Have You Decided What Will Happen to
    Your Life's Work "After You've Gone?" 168

Have a Typewriter Handy So You Can Type
    Your Ideas Out 170

As They Say in Lotto, You Never Know.   172
If You Wanted To Go from New York City to
    Los Angeles, You'd Get a Map!   173
Find Out What You Do Best and Then Train Your
    Brain in Your Strong Points   174
Remember, Your Brain Is the Storeroom for Your Thoughts   176
Feed Things into Your Brain   178
Train Your Brain   179
What Would Keep You Happy in Your Senior Years?   180
What Are You Expecting from Others?   182
Control Your Food Intake   184
If You Have To Be Somewhere at a Certain Time,
    Try To Be There a Little Ahead of Time   186
Don't Sell Yourself Short   188
In America, Everyone Has a Chance   190
You Must Have the Goods   193
Give Yourself a Chance   195
English and Math to Me Are the Two Most Important
    Subjects We Must Study in America   196
"It's Not What You Know, but Who You Know." Total Bull!   198
Do You Get Embarrassed?   200
Do You Pray?   202
You Have a Brain, Use It!   204
Keep Reminding Yourself That You Must Stay on Track.   206
If I Knew at Twenty What I Know at Eighty   208
Have a Second Typewriter As a Backup, Just in Case   210
Are You Jealous of Others?   212
How Do You See Yourself?   213
"Simplicity," Dizzy Gillespie Said to One
    of His Drummers   215
Start at the Age of Fifteen or Sixteen   217
The Amazing Brain   219
More About the Brain   220
Even More About the Brain   222

Introduction

When I finished my book, *I LOVE WHAT I DO! A DRUMMER'S PHILOSOPHY AT EIGHTY*, I was asked by some of my friends why I wrote the book. I always came up with the same answer: IT WAS LIKE A REVELATION. I sat down at my typewriter and the ideas just seemed to pour out of my mind. It was like finding a religion. It just happened that way.

Well, here I am, back with a sequel, and the same thing happened to me again. NEW IDEAS KEPT COMING OUT OF MY MIND AND MY HANDS JUST STARTED TO TYPE. I cannot explain this to you. It just seems to happen. It's almost scary.

The thoughts you will find in this follow-up book can be added to what I wrote about in Book One, perhaps as some form of reinforcement of the original statements I made.

For example, I am a big believer in having a system; in my life, with my work, with my money, with my practicing. There must be a system if we are to get better at what we do. Only with an organized program can we succeed. I don't care who wants to debate this idea, I feel there has to be a real solid method in order to accomplish something in your life.

I always cite this example of why things are successful — take banks, supermarkets, the army, the navy, the federal government, or even a band — all of these businesses are working with a program that someone put together. This is what makes these organizations work. Someone is the head of the organization, the leader, or the director, and this person forms a plan. Many times there is a Board of Directors which helps develop a system. The results depend on whether the system itself is a good one. If the company fails, many times the system has fallen apart. But a good system is necessary to make a company successful.

We may not agree with the way things are done, but there must be a program, and everyone must know what his or her job in that company is.

There Are Twenty-four Hours in a Day

I always say there isn't anything perfect in this world of ours. However, there are two things I think are near-perfect; they are: the days in the year, (three hundred sixty-five, except for leap year), and then the twenty-four hours in a day. These two ideas are as perfect as we can get. At least this is how I see it.

Think of this: If we take a day with twenty-four hours in it and divide it so we can extract the most out of these twenty-four hours, we can accomplish quite a bit. Let's look at the twenty-four-hour day this way: We need sleep. Some of us can get along with eight hours of sleep while others may get along with six. Then, during the day, we may "catnap" for ten or twenty minutes, once or twice a day. It's different for each of us. How do they say? **"DIFFERENT STROKES FOR DIFFERENT FOLKS."** So now we set the amount of time we need for sleep. Each of us will be the judge of how much sleep we require.

Next, we need to schedule time for our toilet duties; to shower, have some breakfast, and plan our day. These things might take an hour every morning. Then we need another hour for lunch and another for supper. Every one of us has a different schedule, but I can get along with a minimum of time for breakfast, lunch, and supper, plus my toilet duties. Now we must decide how much time is free for each of us.

I have lots of free time. I need to practice my instrument, I need time to write new books, or continue whatever I am working on, so for myself, I have my day worked out. Unless I do, I will not get anything done.

So each of us must take each day, one at a time, and use the twenty-four hours to fit our lifestyle. Sounds simple enough, but it's most important that we stick to the schedule we have planned for ourselves. It really works if you set your mind to it. It's not easy, but it can be done.

Over the many years I have been involved with my drums, I have written over two thousand books. I do the hand manuscript and try to do the best I can with the explanation of what the book is about and how a student or educator should use the material in the book. I then have copies made and have the book printed on three-hole paper so it can fit into the folders. I design a cover, make fifty copies of each book to start with, and I'm off and running. Easy? I think so, but when you try it, you'll be surprised at the work involved in making a book.

What I am trying to get across here is that you need to do this within an organized system. This will help you do the things you desire.

Never Feel Sorry for Yourself

I always say that no one else will feel sorry for you, so why feel sorry for yourself? In my mind, I do the best at what I am trying to do. If it turns out well, I am happy. If it turns out not so "hotsy-totsy," I don't feel sorry. At least I know that I have given it my best shot.

Remember that feeling sorry for yourself isn't the answer. Brooding about something that you worked on and getting discouraged that it didn't work out as you had planned and hoped it would doesn't solve the problem. For myself, I never get disappointed in myself. The fact that I tried satisfies me. If it wasn't what I wanted, I'm not ecstatic, but I always feel that I eventually will come up with the answer.

Let me cite a perfect example of why I say this. A while back, I came up with the idea for the first book, called *I LOVE WHAT I DO! A DRUMMER'S PHILOSOPHY AT EIGHTY*. It started out as just an idea. I sat down and completed the book. I then gave it to Ed Petoniak and he did the editing.

Now, mind you, I'm far from being a professional writer, but somehow, quite a few people thought it was a good solid piece of writing. And the next thing I knew, some publishers felt it should be available to the public. I hadn't given that aspect of my writing the slightest thought. Vital Health Publishing/*ENHANCEMENT BOOKS* thought my work was worth publishing, and here I am with a sequel, *KEEP SWINGING!*

I think if I had felt sorry for myself in my life, I would never have done the things I've done and still am doing. Feeling sorry for one's self, or self pity, does not get the job done. You have to do as the song says, "Straighten Up and Fly Right." Give it another effort. Maybe the next time it will come out as you wanted.

Remember this, no one else feels sorry for you. No one else will be crying for you. Crying over spilled milk doesn't solve the problem and you will just make yourself miserable. **WHO NEEDS THAT?**

Plan out what you are going to do. Get advice from people who have been successful and work the problem out. Don't berate yourself. Don't feel sorry for yourself. It doesn't work. Take it from me. At the age of eighty-two, I have learned that feeling bad and disgusted and sorry for yourself isn't how life should be lived.

What do they say? **IF AT FIRST YOU DON'T SUCCEED, TRY UNTIL YOU DO.**

You Can't Spend More Than You Have

It took me a lot of years to learn this very important fact of life: **You can't spend more than you have.** Or, another way to put it is to say you can't spend what you don't have. I remember in my younger days, I did things that always backfired on me. I would buy things with money I was expecting to get. Then things happened and I found myself in a bind. I really hurt myself.

But I eventually learned that all-important fact of life. If you don't have it, you can't spend it. It's as simple as that. I always found that what I wanted to do required dollars, so I saved my money and when I had enough, I bought what I wanted.

I learned that having credit cards wasn't the answer either. It's now over thirty-five years that I haven't had a credit card. When I had credit cards I was always **in debt** and I didn't like it. I made up my mind that I wasn't going to have credit cards and so never hurt myself. What a pleasure; no bills at the end of the month; **No temptation to want to buy things and pay for them later.**

I have a feeling many of us have learned that when you don't have the dollars to do what you wish, you can't do it. **No way.** There are certain bills we need to pay each month: rent, telephone, electricity, maybe a heating or water bill, and perhaps insurance. There are many other needs that have to be met. So you try your best to stay ahead and you feel great when there aren't those bills in your mailbox.

Don't count on money you are expecting to have. Don't spend the dollars that you are thinking will be mailed to you. If checks come in, deposit them and wait until they clear, so you're sure the money is there.

As a young fellow, I always jumped the gun. I paid on expected money, paid on uncleared checks. And then this financial mess would start. I know you want to stay on top of your bucks, but you can't do that with what you haven't received. I have also learned not to make a promise I couldn't keep. Telling so and so, "I'll pay it MONDAY," when I don't have the cash at hand is DANGEROUS to my reputation of dependability.

It's like telling someone you're going to be somewhere at a certain time and arriving late or not showing up at all. YOUR WORD IS MOST IMPORTANT AND YOU MUST LEARN TO KEEP IT.

I've learned these lessons well and now in my later years I have my finances under control and am happy that I can do what I need to do without getting all screwed up. Learn this lesson fast. SPEND ONLY WHAT YOU HAVE.

You Can Only Help Yourself.
Each of Us Must Do It for Ourselves

It's interesting that I learned as I was getting older and developing my talents that no one could do it for me. Only I could do it. I spent a great part of my professional musical life studying and training my brain to learn my craft. I put in as much as ten to fifteen hours a day of hard, serious practice. In fact, at the age of eighty-two, going on eighty-three, I still practice every day about eight to ten hours.

I recall teaching a young chap who was a professional caddy for one of the top professional golfers. This young man said he was an excellent golfer and shot in the low seventies. I asked him why he didn't become one of the top pros? He said he couldn't, because he didn't spend ten or more hours each day, seven days a week on the golf links. All or most of the top professional golfers live this kind of life.

Most professional sports figures — baseball players, boxers, tennis players — spend their lives working at their abilities. They may weight train, bat the ball all day, play games, and constantly work at their professional life in sports. I've often heard it said that it's how it has to be done. When we see the professionals at their game, we see the tops, because these people spend their lives training and developing their talents.

I made up my mind as a young man to study hard, practice, read books, write books, listen to the professionals, and listen to the melody player who could direct me. I studied the books and practiced over and over and over until I knew what I was doing. Even when I sit here and type, I have the radio playing, Latin music, jazz, commercials, or rock, to try to see if I can cover all the bases I have to in my studies. I do this for myself because, as I said, NO ONE ELSE WILL DO IT FOR ME.

This is how I see it. When we learn this and can work at improving our abilities, we'll find we alone can do what has to be done. When we're children, Mom and Pop will direct us, teach us, and help us mature. Then, when we have developed as a grown-up, we will have to make our own living, support ourselves, save our dollars, and all the rest as we advance in our lives. Some never learn this lesson and still depend on parents, wives, or children. Then this becomes a problem.

Think about this: We find what we like and love to do and now we must go after the results. It takes hours, years of hard work to develop as a professional, whether it's as a doctor, lawyer, educator, or politician, but once we decide what we want to be and want to do with our lives, each of us must seek the information and training to become our own selves.

There Is Always a Way To Do Something Better

I'm a big believer that there is always a way to do something better. In my early days as a young student of the drums, I knew that there had to be a better way to learn my instrument. I know that sounds strange, but as the years rolled by, I searched until I discovered a better method to improve my talents. I studied with over forty instructors until I found someone who could explain and demonstrate for me what I needed to know.

Of course I practiced constantly. Through trial and error, I eventually worked out the problems until I learned my craft. Many of my educators stopped practicing and as they got older, these teachers couldn't play any longer. I spent hours and hours until I found what I was searching for and eventually it came to me.

As the song would say, "THERE MUST BE A WAY," and sure enough there was!

There aren't any shortcuts. There are no simple solutions to finding what works. I think once we learn that lesson, we are on the right track. When I was confronted with a problem, I would write a book covering that particular hurdle. I practiced the material I wrote about. I found the answers.

If you get discouraged and give up, you can't find the key to what you were trying to work out. But if you work at it and study the problem, I am certain you will find the right method. I knew it could be done. I knew I was working the kinks out of my drumming ideas.

Although many of my educators had no answers to certain questions, I came up with them. If you practice, if you study the situation, you will find your answers. I did, so why can't you? Pay your dues and you'll get the payoff. Believe me. It is true.

As the Song Says, "Pick Yourself Up and Start All Over Again"

I always liked the title of this song. It is so true. We must all learn how to do this. When you fall, you just pick yourself up and start all over again. It's a great statement and makes a lot of sense. I have learned over these many years that if I'm working on something and it fails or doesn't come out as I had expected, I give it a second try. I go back to the beginning and see if I can work the problems out. Sometimes it works and sometimes I need to change things.

Getting discouraged and chucking the plan isn't an answer. I step back and look at what I have done up to this point and ask myself if what I'm doing is how I feel it should be done? Sometimes just taking another look gives me the answer. Sometimes I lay the material down and give it a few days to work itself out in my mind. Many times I eventually find the answer and then can complete what I am working on. I always take my material seriously until I do.

As we get older, our minds and brains find a method to complete what we started. I have many instruction books that I began quite a few years ago. All of a sudden, something pops and I discover how I wanted to complete a certain project I was developing. No kidding! It's so interesting to me how this works itself out.

When I was about fifteen years old, I wrote some of my first drum instruction books and years later I published them. Some of these study books are still in print. When I wrote those beginning books, I had no idea what I was going to do with them. As I learned my instrument and understood why I wrote these studies, I realized I should publish these books and they've been used in the music industry for many years.

I'm a big believer that there isn't anything that can be called a failure. I'm certain many great composers and artists have been disappointed with what would later be called some of their best work. Maybe they didn't see it at first, but eventually they recognized that what looked like a failed effort really wasn't. Sometimes our inexperience doesn't allow us to understand what we have accomplished.

So if you fail, or think what you've done is a failure, perhaps later on you'll see that you did something worthwhile and eventually see it wasn't a failure. You can then turn it into a success. So, as the song says, **"PICK YOURSELF UP AND START ALL OVER AGAIN."** If at first you don't succeed...

Have You Made Up Your Mind As to What You Love To Do?

As young people, many of us hadn't decided what we would love to do. When I was teaching at the summer camps at Elon College in North Carolina, Professor Jack O. White used to say: "YOU HAVE TO LOVE YOUR INSTRUMENT, YOU HAVE TO LOVE TO PRACTICE," and "YOU HAVE TO LOVE YOUR MUSIC." (I remember his heavy southern accent.) Professor White would tell his students, "You have to love what you want to do in your life."

Now, many years later, I really understand what he was talking about. You must love what you do so much that you can almost taste it. The love of life and music and your musical instrument has to be in your brain and your gut. Professor White loved to conduct and practice and play his trumpet. He had a running love affair with his love for music and tried hard to pass this on to all of his students. I agree with him totally.

I think had I not loved what I do I might not have reached the point in my life where I became inspired to write about my Philosophy of Life. Now, at eighty-two, I really understand what making my mind up means to me.

Liking what you do, to me, is not sufficient. I want to do only what I love. This way I can work day after day at my inner joy. It's so important to me. I have many friends who just spend day after day searching for that one thing that would give them the inner glow that comes from doing what you love to do. It's not easy to find, but it's there and when we recognize it, we know we've found our greatest desire.

Make up your mind about what you love to do and give it a shot. If you find it's not what you really wanted to do in your life, then search some more. Maybe the next time it will show up and you might find that which you love.

I think I am one of the lucky ones, because I discovered my love for drums and music at a very early age. Along with my love for the instrument, I found that I love to practice, write, play, lecture, and teach. The next thing I had to do was to follow the dream in my heart. It's a wonderful feeling to know that you have found what you love to do. **AND DO IT UNTIL YOU CAN DO IT CONSISTENTLY.**

Do You Change Your Mind Often?

A s I have said so many times, I feel I am one of the lucky ones who found what I love and have stayed with it all of these years. SOON I WILL BE PLAYING AND ENJOYING DRUMS FOR NEARLY SEVENTY YEARS. I don't know too many people who can honestly say that they have found their heart's desire and have been doing it all of their lives!

Just think how fortunate you would be if you could find what you love to do and are able to do it all of your life. When you discover what you love, you will understand that it will take years to develop and YEARS OF STUDY AND STAYING ON TOP OF YOUR GAME. This is the secret of life as I see it.

Keep in mind that what I'm writing about doesn't work for all of us. Maybe it will for a few, however. If and when you recognize what you are searching for and find it, then stick with it. Changing your mind very often can be a problem. If you change your mind often about what to do with your life, it can make you unhappy and cause you lots of trouble.

As the song says, "First you say you will and then you won't. Then you say you do and then you don't. You're undecided now. What are you gonna do?" Not a very good way to live your life. I would go "bananas" if I lived my life that way. Such disruption. Not very good. Going left and then going right because you can't make up your mind can be so painful.

Of course, when we are young, we really don't know what we want out of life. There are people who never find out. But somewhere along the way, most of us find ourselves. When you do, I believe that you will know it. It will jump up and kick you in the face. You'll know it in your heart and mind. That's what I think.

Someone once asked me, if I had my life to live over again, would I have done it differently? I said I would do it exactly the same way. I love what I have done all of my life and I know of nothing else that would have given me the joy and satisfaction that I have gained from the work I do.

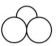

Are You Flexible?

Over the past years of my musical life as a professional drummer, I have learned that I am able to be flexible. Knowing this about myself has allowed me to Go WITH THE FLOW, so to speak.

Being rigid can be a hang-up because there are times we must be able to bend. I've watched many friends in my field be inflexible. If they were in the Broadway scene, that was all they could do. Those who were in the Dixieland field played that style and could not play in the Latin, Bebop styles, or many of the other styles that were developing.

I am a big believer that we must be able to bend and play in as many styles as possible. I've learned to teach, write, lecture, and perform in a great many musical situations. This meant that I could be working most of the time. That is a good way to be, I think. It allowed me to travel in many musical circles. I play the jazz field and the wedding and bar mitzvah scene. I can produce my own recordings and I am able to market what I produce.

It's good to be a specialist in your field, but you must have other irons in the fire. I remember Henny Youngman, the great comedian, who said his mother wanted him to learn a trade so at least she would know what kind of work he was out of. My family always wanted me to know more than drumming and as I look back now, my mom was right. She felt we should learn as much as we could so we could bend with the changes and be able to travel in the many areas of whatever field we chose. My mother was very wise. All of my brothers and sisters could do many things and always were able to survive in this world of ours.

Train yourself to be flexible. Be able to change directions and do more than just one thing. I write books and I market them, I teach drummers and try to give them the wider picture about being a drummer. I tell all my students to teach and play in order to be the best they can be in their profession. Not only do my students learn to play their instrument, but they learn to move in many directions.

Think about this: If you are a band player and that's all you can do and the bands you work with have a dry spell, you've got no work. What do you do for income? But if you teach and have twenty or so students and your band is out of work, you still can make a dollar to support yourself. It's very important that you have what we call "cash flow," so that you at least can keep going. Then, when work with bands comes in, you are still able to keep your head above water.

BE FLEXIBLE. BE ABLE TO BEND. HAVE MORE THAN ONE EGG IN YOUR BASKET.

Do You Care for What You Do?

One of my former teachers used to say to me, "You must care for what you do." No matter what it might be, you must care for what you are trying to do with your life. When I started to play the drums as a young person, I knew right then that it was what I wanted to do. I wanted to play the drums. I cared for my study (and I was very serious about it) even at the age of thirteen.

All during my life my educators would say that you have to contribute as much time as possible to your study work. In the long run, they said, you'll see the results of the hours you put into training yourself. Now at age eighty-two, I do see the results and I'm so happy with what I did all those years.

If you don't care for what you do, you are wasting your time and your life. Life is too short to let it pass you by. Think of this when you wake up and say to yourself, "What will I do with these beautiful twenty-four hours? What do I want to do with my life?"

You must make decisions about the direction you want to take. You must care for what you want to do with your life. The sooner you know what you are after and how you wish to develop the talent the LORD gave you, the sooner you are on the right track.

In place of the word "care" or "caring," I use the word LOVE — do what you love to do with your life. Loving and caring go together. If you care enough and love it enough, you will get great satisfaction from the time you put into growing in your chosen field.

If you don't care, then it's not worth much. When you succeed, you will see how loving and caring about what you are doing pays off. I have found, with the study and practice I put into developing my skills, if you care, you will see the final results of your abilities — and that's what it is all about.

While I am writing my philosophy of life, I care about it a great deal, because I might give the reader some ideas that he or she didn't have before reading what I have to say. I might give readers reasons to care and put them on the right track. At least I hope so. This is why I care about what I am writing. I might just make you care also, AS MUCH AS I CARE.

Does the Weather Affect Your Daily Life?

Many times I hear people say that the weather has an effect on their everyday life. I must be a strange duck, because I am not affected one bit by what the weather conditions are outside. Some of my friends say when it's rainy, they feel gloomy. Others tell me that when it's hot outside, they have a problem with feeling like doing something.

I sort of "roll with the punches." I'm happy most of the time. If I feel that I am not working on all cylinders, I ask myself, "What's wrong?" However, I let it roll by and try to "do my thing" that day. I don't feel sorry for myself. I don't feel miserable. I try to stay on top of my game and do some work that is important to me at that time.

I have set goals for myself and I try to complete those goals. It's important for me. I feel I want to be ready for unexpected things. I know this always sounds nutty and crazy to people who know me. However, I would be disappointed in myself if I let things slide.

I practice my drums every day. I do a certain amount of writing every day. If I write just one page a day, I have progressed on a project I am working on. Perhaps it's a new drum study book. Maybe it's something to do with this particular book.

I can't speak for others, only for myself. When I get a specific thing done, I am satisfied with myself. It's a wonderful feeling to know that I have completed what I started.

Think about this: It doesn't matter whether it's homework to be done, letters to write, telephone calls to make, or bills to pay. Whatever it may be, it's great to know that you have completed what you had to complete that day.

I never let the weather affect my mental health. I don't care if it rains, snows, is hot or cold. Weather doesn't control what my minds wants to do. If it bothers you, I think there is something wrong with you. The fact is, I can't do anything about the weather. The old joke is: It's raining outside. I always answer, "As long as it's not raining inside, what should I care?"

I've heard others say that after an operation, rain or hot weather affects them. I have had a number of serious operations on my body over the years and the weather has never affected me. As the television show said, I take it ONE DAY AT A TIME. That's how I face my life. I don't care about the weather. I don't let it bother me. I have too much fun in my life to worry about something I can't control. I roll with the flow.

Do You Learn Something New Every Day?

What a good question! I try to learn something new every day. When I was a youngster, I never paid much attention to learning and so as I got older, I found I knew very little . . . very little about life, sex, money, history, spelling, the world, politics, how to pay my bills . . . thousands of other things. As I got older and became a drum instructor, I realized I didn't speak too well. My English was awful. My concept of life was poor. When I got drafted and played with the U.S. Army Band, I started to understand I was not as educated about things as I thought I was.

I was a serious student as a young man. I had my first drum studio around the age of seventeen, and I knew I had the ability to teach others, but that's all I knew. I recall an experience with the father of a young chap who came to me and wanted to study drums. It turned out to be a great learning experience for me.

The father and his young son came to my studio and wanted to watch me teach. I felt great. I had about twenty or more students. My lesson time lasted about an hour, maybe more. I was finishing with a student as this parent and his son watched me.

The father seemed very impressed with my drum teaching abilities. After I finished with my student, I spoke with this potential new student. Wonderful, I thought. The boy's father said that he thought I showed signs of being a good, qualified teacher. "However, despite the fact that I like your approach to teaching drums, I WILL NOT ALLOW MY SON TO STUDY WITH YOU."

"What's wrong?" I asked. Then the father said to me, "I will not allow my son to study with you because if he learns to speak like you, I would be very unhappy." Then he added that I should learn how to speak English correctly. With that, the father and his son left.

I learned a great deal from that experience and I made certain I would not allow this to happen again. I lost the student, but I gained from what the father said to me. I made up my mind to learn to speak English more correctly.

That's how I started learning something new every day of my life. Even now, at eighty-two, I'm still learning. I want to be the best I can be, not only in playing my instrument, but in how I handle my daily life. I WANT TO GET BETTER.

One of the most important things I have learned is that I don't know everything and can't know everything. So I want to get as good as I can and know my craft and improve my speaking and writing to get myself ready for whatever might happen on a day-to-day basis.

LEARN SOMETHING NEW EACH DAY. This philosophy has helped me in my work as a drummer, as a writer, and as a person.

Do You Go Back on What You Say You Will Do?

This is important to me. I try to stick to what I tell people I will do. Again I go back to my youth. I made up my mind that if I say I will do a certain thing, I will try my best to do it. It's one of my codes, or rules. I don't care that others may say they'll do something and then don't do it. For me, **I STICK TO MY WORD**.

I didn't do that when I was young. I didn't lie to people or to myself, but somewhere along the line I realized I would say that I was going to do a certain thing and I didn't keep my word. That was an important lesson I had to learn in life.

I have had students tell me that they are playing on a certain night, and I find that my student was making up stories about how busy he was. The one who suffers here is the student. When asked for a recommendation, I may not recommend him or her again because I have lost confidence in what was said to me. Know what I mean?

Try not to say things because you want to impress others by making yourself look like a big shot. Tell it like it is and in the long run this can work out to your own good.

If I say something to someone, I will never go back on my word. I do what I say I will do and never change my story. Many times a student will say that he was given a band job and then got another offer, maybe for more money and then he called the first band leader and tried to cancel out of his original obligation. Not a good practice. I did that once, when I was young, and the person never forgave me for going back on my word.

Since then, if I say I will play at a certain function, I keep my word. Many times I might make a few dollars less, but I feel good about myself that I did what I said I was going to do.

Don't say you're going left and then go right. Don't say you will be at your dentist's office and find some excuse to cancel at the last minute. Stick to what you say you'll do. As the years go on, people will know that you are a person whose word can be trusted.

I know there are circumstances when things happen and we can't keep our word, but these are the exceptions. DON'T GO BACK ON YOUR WORD. As they say, "YOU'LL BE SORRY." Take it from me.

Make Rules for Yourself

This is a good idea. At least I have found this to be so. I have a set of rules that I try to live by. Yes, I know this sounds rigid, but in reality it's not. Everyone has a different set of rules or standards that they live by. My rules are not the same as yours. My concept of life is not the same as everyone else's. As they say, "DIFFERENT STROKES FOR DIFFERENT FOLKS."

Men and women may have different levels, rules, or ideas that they live by. Even in our own family, we each have to set individual goals for living our lives. Our goals may be different goals than our siblings and mother and father have.

Sure, there are basics we all live by. Every religion and Bible have pretty much the same standards. DO NOT KILL, DO NOT STEAL, DO NOT TRY TO TAKE ANOTHER'S LOVER FROM THEM, etc. I am certain many of us have read the Bible. This book of laws, rules, and standards sets the bar for all of us. Some of us lose our way and don't stick to these ideas and so we suffer as our life moves on.

Here is an idea of the kinds of rules I make for myself. Remember, these rules are not for everybody. They are for me, Sam Ulano. I have been making lists like this for years. I can't say if it will work for you; however, you might try these ideas and see.

1. Try and get enough sleep.
2. Find a system of exercise that works for you.
3. Make an effort to dress nicely every day.
4. Take care of your eyes. If you need glasses, get them, and use them.
5. Take good care of your legs. To me, this is so important.
6. Don't always be so sure of yourself.
7. Study hard so you know your craft.
8. Don't do things you are not so sure of.
9. Control your money.

10. Try to think ahead at all times.
11. Be ready for the next day.
12. See your doctor and dentist at least twice a year.
13. Don't be conceited.
14. Be confident.
15. Study with the right people for you.
16. As the song says, "You're nobody 'til somebody loves you."
17. If you can't remember your daily schedule, carry a book. Make a list of your daily appointments.
18. If you drive a car: Have two or three sets of keys with you at all times. (The same for your keys for your home.) Keep important papers in the glove compartment at all times. Make sure your insurance is always paid up and covers you and your car properly.
19. Try not to repeat the same mistakes over and over.
20. Try to check your list every day. Add some new rules every day and get rid of the rules that don't work.
21. If you can have a few good friends, maybe you can exchange your rule list with your buddies.
22. When you leave your home, make sure you have your money, keys, special papers you might need, and the list of what you have to do.
23. If you have a cell phone, make sure you have it with you at all times.

I can't tell you what to do and you can't tell others what to do. These ideas work for me. These are some general ideas about how I make my list for myself. It's handy and helps me. It could help you if you give it a try.

Who Are You and Who Do You Want To Be?

To me, this is interesting, because I will be eighty-three on August 12, 2003, and have given this question a great deal of thought. Many of us have a problem with trying to find a place in this marvelous world of ours. I know that I have twenty-four hours in a day to decide who I am and who I want to be.

I know for sure that I want to be me and I found out very quickly in my life who I am. At an early age I knew I wanted to play the drums. When I was going to James Monroe High School in the Bronx, New York, I started to teach other drummers.

This was during the Depression. Money was scarce. I somehow had a feeling that I could teach others. My band director, Mr. Irving Firestein, gave me ten students to teach in school. I was doing well and so I set up a drum studio in my apartment and started to teach for fifty cents a lesson. I even started to write some of my first drum instruction books, charging a dollar to my students.

I found that I enjoyed this, so right then and there I knew that PLAYING THE DRUMS, TEACHING THE DRUMS, AND WRITING ABOUT THE DRUMS was what I wanted to do.

Of course I knew my shortcomings. I too was a beginner and I had practically no real life experience. However, I believed in myself and knew inside of me that I would eventually get this much-needed experience. I knew I could play the instrument, and with hard study and practice I eventually would reach my goal of becoming an educator.

I knew then and there WHO I wanted to be and WHO I WAS. Many of my young friends never knew who they were and what they were going to do with their lives. I was fortunate to discover this about myself at a young age. It came to me like a revelation, like someone finding a gold mine. I didn't make a lot of dollars in the beginning, but I knew I could make a very good living being in many areas of music.

I now know I was right and I know the track I got on was true. The main thing I wanted to be was MYSELF. No one else. I'm still following this fantastic dream and will continue for the rest of my life, wherever it may lead me.

What Is My Idea on How To Become an "Original?"

Many times my students would ask how I think someone can become original. How can someone find and be themselves? I always gave the same answer: JUST BE YOURSELF AND DON'T TRY TO BE SOMEONE ELSE.

Someone once said that imitation was the greatest form of flattery. I've always said that the same energy one puts into imitation can be put into being original. Or, as I've heard for years, amateurs teach amateurs to be amateurs; PROFESSIONALS TEACH PROFESSIONALS TO BE PROFESSIONAL.

Why put your time into trying to be someone else? Why not put your time into finding yourself? That is what I wanted from my life. I would say to myself: "SAM, BE SAM AND NO ONE ELSE." Why would someone want to imitate someone else? Why not search for who you are?

As the song says, "I WANT TO BE ME." I would become very annoyed when someone would come over to me and say, "YOU SOUND LIKE GENE KRUPA," (or BUDDY RICH, or whomever). Find your own identity. Look into yourself and see if you can be yourself and follow that path.

Over the years I write my books in my style and I write about subjects in my field that I feel have not yet been covered. I noticed over the years so much about drumming that had not been documented. I followed that out to the end and have created many of the most original books in the field. My style. My concept.

If that sounds like I'm blowing my own horn, so be it. If someone doesn't like it, then that is their problem. I must be me and no one else. I would be very disappointed in myself if I was copying what others did.

Think about this: Ella Fitzgerald had her own sound; Sarah Vaughn had her own sound and style; Sinatra had his distinct sound and concept. Bing Crosby had his sound. Benny, Dizzy, Max Roach, Buddy Rich, Harry James, Miles Davis, Tony Bennett, Bobby Darin, and so many other great stars did. All had their own unique sound and style. That's what made them so beautiful.

I listen to everybody but I try to be myself. ORIGINAL SAM IS WHAT I WANTED IN MY LIFE. I WOULDN'T SETTLE FOR ANYTHING LESS.

So I say to my students and friends, FIND YOURSELF AND WHO YOU ARE AND BE WHO YOU ARE . . . NO ONE ELSE.

The search goes on for each of us. Be who you are and you'll enjoy your life always. TAKE IT FROM ME . . . I have learned this, and it is what has made me completely happy. NOTHING ELSE CAN OR WILL.

You Have To Work at Staying in Top Physical Shape Like an Athlete

In my first book I wrote about finding a method of keeping your body in the best physical shape that you can. Again I remind you that this is one of the keys of living well and finding some happiness in your existence. I now can really make a definitive statement on this topic because I've learned my lesson well. It has been the key to my loving what I do and it has helped me come up with my philosophy of life. It works for me; maybe not for others, but for me.

I pass this concept on to my students and many friends in fields other than music. Staying in the best physical shape you can is so important. You will find this out as you grow older and eventually come to the same conclusion that I have.

I see it with myself. When I think I'll soon be eighty-three years old, it's interesting to think of how the years fly by. In my early years, I knew nothing about staying in shape. I heard a lot about it, read articles, saw health and body conditioning magazines on the newsstands. I saw it on television and heard many people talking about it. When I got into the ARMY BAND in 1942, I weighed one hundred fifty-four pounds and was in wonderful shape. I did no body exercise. The ARMY taught me a great deal about staying in shape through RUNNING, HIKING, SWIMMING, WALKING. The whole bit. But it still never struck home in my COMPUTER BRAIN.

I got out of the Army in 1946, got married, had a son and daughter. I was then forty years old (1960) and weighed three hundred twenty pounds. Then I met SIGMOND KLEIN. He was the man who taught me what body conditioning was all about. I learned my lesson well. These past years I have been preaching good health and body conditioning to all who meet me: to students, other educators, friends, the entire gang.

I tell everybody to find a way to stay in shape and stick to it. My favorite line is: **"IF YOU DON'T, YOU'LL BE SORRY."** Many have been sorry, suffering with all kinds of problems. When I see fat people walking the streets, on the bus, wherever I play, I want to tell everyone that they are heading for a body crash, but it wouldn't do any good. **THE SWITCH IN OUR BRAIN MUST BE TURNED ON.** Then and only then will it strike home.

We must find a system to retrain our bodies. Books and magazines can't do it for us. **WE MUST DO THIS FOR OURSELVES.** Like an athlete, you must train your body.

There Aren't Any Shortcuts

When I started to retrain my body I asked Sigmond Klein, "Are there any shortcuts to getting back into shape?" He asked me HOW LONG IT TOOK FOR ME TO GET TO THREE HUNDRED TWENTY POUNDS AND OUT OF SHAPE? I replied that it took me twenty-five years. Klein shot back to me, "Well, Sam, it will take you twenty-five years to rehabilitate your body. You just have to reverse what you were doing and you will eventually get back in shape."

He was saying it took twenty-five years to get out of shape and now will take twenty-five years to get myself back into shape. You want to know something? HE WAS RIGHT. I am now forty-two years into my system of rehabilitating my body and I am almost completely back to where I was when I started to let myself deteriorate into the fat slob I was. Makes sense, doesn't it? To me it does, and unless we think this way we never will find a way back.

In other words, Klein was saying to me and others that there aren't any shortcuts. No Ten-Day Diet. No losing thirty pounds in a month. No "quick" method to being what we were when we allowed ourselves to fall apart and become overweight. There's just no fast system to return to the wonderful shape we were in years ago.

Let's not kid ourselves, everybody. You must first become aware of what this body of ours is all about. We get only one life, one chance, one crack at keeping it brand new. Do you know what I mean?

THINK, THINK, THINK. First we are young. We get a little older, into our twenties and may fall in love, get married, buy a house, have kids, and raise our family. Here's when we tend to overeat: at our home, on holidays like Thanksgiving, Passover, Christmas; birthday and wedding celebrations. EAT, EAT, EAT. We eat the wrong foods, or should I say too much food. We eat before we go to bed, eat a big breakfast, lunch, supper. We snack while watching television, go to bed on a full stomach, OVEREAT ALL THE TIME. We overeat in restaurants, at the movies, things like candy, chocolate, pizza, hamburgers, fast food . . . I FEEL LIKE I WANT TO THROW UP. No control.

There are NO SHORTCUTS. On top of all of this eating, we tend to drink too much beer and wine at parties, on New Year's Eve, baby births, and so on. What can I tell you?

The picture I'm painting I went through, except that I never drank and stopped smoking many years ago. I began to watch my diet, and eliminated a lot of what I was eating. Sounds boring, but I'm in great shape and happily alive. So keep in mind, THERE ARE NO SHORTCUTS TO STAYING WELL AND ALIVE. It's up to you.

I Believe You Must Get Your Inspiration from Within Yourself

Someone once asked me what or who inspires me? I said, "I get my inspiration from within myself. I get it from **GOD**, the **LORD**."

I really don't know, exactly. However, I am a big believer in the **LORD**. I am Jewish and I believe there is a Power that is bigger than all of us. I don't know if it's **GOD**. I like to think there is a **GOD** over all of us. For myself, I believe there is something watching over **SAM ULANO**. I don't know where this feeling comes from, but this seems to be where I get the idea that inspiration in my daily existence comes from what I conceive as **GOD**, a Supreme Power.

I wake up and I have all these ideas gushing out of my brain. As you know, I consider the brain to be the greatest computer. I had mentioned this in the first book, *I LOVE WHAT I DO*. This is how my Philosophy of Life at Eighty developed. What gave me the inspiration to put pen to paper? I really do not know. I can't give you an answer.

I saw this concept one morning about 3:00A.M. I got up to go to the bathroom and as I got back into bed, I jumped up and took out my writing pad and started writing the concept of how I saw the first book and how I would write it and what I wanted to say. It's as simple as all that.

Now, I envisioned a second book of my Philosophy of Life at eighty-two. Again, I can't explain why this came to me, but again I have this feeling that I am driven to this concept. That "something," some Power called me to the pen and pad and I saw all these ideas and topics that I could write about. And so, here it is!

I feel that I have this ability to motivate myself to write my thoughts and then try to expand on each of these ideas. Go figure it out. I can't. I love to teach, I love what I do, and I love to explain and write about these things.

All of my life, even as a young person, this ability to write my ideas just seemed to flow like good wine out of my brain into my hands. I really feel inspired and what sets off this desire to write and document this concept of my life just seems to happen. I can be sleeping at night and wake up and the switch in my brain just goes on LIKE A LIGHT BULB. Ideas just pour out of my head.

I imagine this is like when someone writes a song, a Broadway show, a book, a film. How we create has always been a mystery to me. This is called talent. Some call it a "calling," others call it our imagination. I can't explain it to you. I just know I inspire myself. I need no one else to inspire me. Maybe I was inspired by something that might have happened to me in the past and didn't know it. Then, all of a sudden, it happens and I'm inspired. Silly, ain't it?

Wishing Is Nice, but It Doesn't Work

"WHEN YOU WISH UPON A STAR . . ." is very nice, but I often wonder about this wishing thing. The little fellow is asking GOD if He will let him win the Lotto just this one time and he'd never bother GOD again. He says, "I wish you would allow me to win the Lotto just this once" and GOD says to this fellow, "It's a good idea, but instead of wishing, go buy a ticket."

We make a wish when we blow out the candles on a birthday cake. We dream and wish and hope and pray for our wishes to come true. It's nice, but I think we need to go into action and do the work to make things happen in our life. Wishing is fun and I don't want to burst our bubbles, but we must do the work that will lead to our wishes coming true. Preparation and study and hard work are what makes things come true.

I believe in doing the work and "paying the dues" to make our dreams and wishes come true for us. Try to do the studying. Try to learn how to read and how to play with a band. Study every day so you are ready for the opportunities that may come. You can wish all you want, every night, every year, it will not work, my friend. Take care of your body, learn your craft, and be ready for your opportunity when it happens. I believe if we work hard and know what we are doing, we can make all of our wishes come true. In reality, it was not wishing that made things happen, it was hard work.

Some of us are superstitious. Some of us believe in fortune-tellers. Some of us close our eyes and wish real hard. I am realistic and I know that it is not the reason things happen in our lives. STUDY HARD EVERY DAY. PRACTICE HARD EVERY DAY. GO TO COLLEGE AND DO THE WORK NEEDED TO MAKE YOU THE BEST YOU CAN BE. THIS WILL HELP YOUR DREAMS AND WISHES COME ABOUT.

If you believe in fantasies or in fairy tales, put a piece of cake under your pillow to make your wishes come true. IT'S NOT

GOING TO HAPPEN. Do not be disappointed if your wishes don't materialize. Don't get your hopes up with wishes.

BE REAL. LIVE YOUR LIFE AND WISH, BUT DO THAT WITH TONGUE IN CHEEK. NOTHING COMES EASY. NOTHING IS EVER BUILT ON A WISH, THAT'S FOR CHILDREN, NOT ADULTS. It's very beautiful, but not as beautiful as the real thing.

Just a Reminder:
Your Health Is Most Important

You probably wonder why I stress taking care of our health. Every month or so I have to be at the VETERAN'S HOSPITAL, here in New York City. As a diabetic and someone who takes special medication, I find myself reminded how much of our lives depend upon making sure we are in tip-top shape. As we get older it becomes more apparent that we should keep this uppermost in our minds: GOOD HEALTH GIVES US A BETTER CHANCE TO BE ABLE TO DO OUR BEST.

One thing I missed out on in my growing years was understanding how to stay in shape, how to eat the right foods, and how to train my body. No one in my family and none of my friends then knew anything about how important body conditioning was and why we should be made aware of it. None of my drum instructors knew anything about this phase of our training as a drummer. None of my schoolteachers talked about or explained why good body development was essential to our daily lifestyle.

My instructors themselves were overweight and out of condition. They didn't know anything about what one should do to keep the body strong and in the best physical shape for playing the drums. They couldn't tell their students why it was necessary to develop strong bodies, strong legs, stomach, and back.

Because my teachers didn't know anything about body development, I and all my fellow students suffered from lack of knowledge about this type of training. As I got to age forty, one of my own students explained body workouts to me and took me to Sigmond Klein's gym. I've written quite a bit about this over the years.

The last forty plus years of my life have been wonderful because I stuck to the program that Klein planned for me. I must say that this was the most important part of my life as I grew older, and having my arms, legs, back, shoulders, stomach, the complete body in good solid condition has paid off for me.

So I remind you that finding a system that works for you to help you stay in the best physical shape is a most important part of living. Once you do this in a regular routine, you can do all of the other things that you want to do in your life: your daily job, taking care of your family, enjoying every holiday, participating in sports, dancing, and enjoying your food.

Staying in shape can cut down the amount of physical ailments we go through during our lives too!

Take it from me, you'll enjoy the payoff in the long run.

Have Patience in Whatever You Do

Nothing comes fast. Nothing should be done in a hurry. Everything you plan to do should be sketched out on paper and in your mind. Think it out clearly and take it step by step. I've found that by learning something slowly at first, I was able to develop what I wanted to do and, little by little, I saw great results.

Somewhere I've heard or read that haste makes waste. It is definitely so. Anytime I do something too fast, I always have terrible results. Nothing works out as it should.

I have an interesting method that I use in teaching my students the ability to learn to read drum music. I tell them to think of a SLOW-MOTION CAMERA. You slow up what you want to do and practice it as slowly as you can. Let your brain and mind absorb the ideas you are working with. GO SLOWLY AT FIRST.

Then, as you know what you are doing, try to do it just a bit faster. The slow-motion camera allows you to break down at a slow pace what you are trying to learn. Gradually you do it a bit faster. Go back to slow again and now that you know it better, pick up the speed and do it faster.

As I learned the keyboard of the typewriter, I gradually developed the skill to type faster. I still type in what is known as the "hunt and peck" style, with one finger of each hand. However, I can do it quite rapidly. I've become quite an expert at typing in my style and system. I couldn't be a secretary in an office, but when I want to write my own ideas down, I can type two fingers style very fast. I started slowly many years ago and now I call myself a professional. Well, sort of.

Having patience is really important. Take your time. Work at a snail's pace. Do that for weeks and months. Eventually you'll accomplish quite a bit. This can happen in anything you wish to do.

In my teaching, I have all my students play slowly at first. If they try to play faster than their eyes can scan the material, they will stumble and fumble all over the place. Fast doesn't work and you should know that right from the start. Give yourself a chance to learn what you want to learn with control and patience.

At eighty-two I have learned my lesson well. I've written many books in the past months doing a few pages at a time. I write every day. At the end I have completed what I started out to do. Sounds easy, doesn't it? It really isn't as simple as I make it sound, but once you have developed the patience, then it's a snap. YOU'LL SEE.

You Can't Discuss or Give an Opinion on a Subject About Which You Know Nothing

As American citizens, we all can have an opinion about any topic. However, I've always believed that we really can't talk about a subject if we really don't know much about it. I know about drumming — the study, the music, and the application — because that is what I have been involved with most of my life. I have studied, practiced, and developed my talents in this field, so I feel I know a great deal about percussion.

I know a little about a lot of things, but there are things I know very little about. I wouldn't call myself an authority on any of these subjects. Thus I keep my mouth shut when I hear others talk about what they know. Capisci? Farshteyt? (Do you understand?)

Now that I have lived this long, it seems I became smarter in my later life. I let others do the talking and I learn so much by listening. I'll ask questions and be part of the conversation, but mostly as a person trying to learn.

I never tell a woman how she should do things that women generally know about and men generally don't. This is helpful advice when you're with your wife, girlfriend, or a group of ladies. A man can sound so stupid trying to tell the other sex about things that women know best.

I get a kick out of hearing others discuss the music world when they are not involved in it. They might be good listeners but they know nothing about the inner workings of being a musician.

The drum is the second oldest instrument known to man, but very few people dedicate themselves to a disciplined study of drums and to understanding what makes the drums "tick."

46

Every so often I'm told things about drums by people who know nothing about drums. They sound so silly and I must tell them that they know nothing when it comes to drumming. I have to say something because it bugs me that people like to sound like they are an authority on the subject. How can someone make statements about things they are not involved with and which aren't their area of expertise? That just doesn't work for me.

Quite often I am with relatives or friends and they tell me things about music that they saw on television. They quote these television shows as authoritative about music. Recently there was a series of programs on TV dealing with JAZZ and the history of jazz. It was a very one-sided series of films and wasn't accurate about the subject. The people who put it together just didn't know what was so.

I've lived through many years of music and many phases of the music scene. I also have been in music all of my life, yet I still do not consider myself a "maven" about the subject. And I say so!

If You Are Going for an Interview, Make Sure You Are Totally Prepared

In the eighty-two years I've lived, I have learned a great lesson: I must be ready at all times for whatever may come. For instance, I was interviewed by one of the better drum publications, STICK IT magazine, and the interviewer was Mark Griffith. The editor is known in the percussion field as ZORO.

I had all my material ready: bios, photos, past articles about me, and other pieces of information that I thought might be of value to the interview. I brought copies of my CDs and audio cassettes and copies of a few of the many instruction books I wrote and published.

Keep in mind when you do an interview that you are the person that has to feed information to the interviewer. This person may have an idea of who you are, but you have to fill in the blanks about what you do, what you've done in the past, and what you plan for the future. You are the one who knows this best.

Don't be too modest. Don't be afraid to let out what you want the interviewer to know about you. Have as much material ready as possible. Dress nicely because the interviewer might take some photographs of you or might bring a photographer along. Always look professional. Look "adult" and clean. That's my concept of this type of thing.

The interviewer is looking for something interesting about you in order to build a story. You might talk about something humorous in your life, something about your past, and, if you are a performer, where you will be appearing. Then you might add a lot of general ideas about yourself.

I always say, I know me. The same goes for you. You know you. That's why you are the one who has to supply the material for an interesting article.

If you are going for a job interview, it will be similar to what I have said, only this will be a live, one-on-one interview for a specific position. Again, you must present yourself as professionally as possible. FIRST IMPRESSIONS ARE IMPORTANT.

Listen and Learn

In my early life, one of my teachers always said that we should learn something new every day of our lives. Somehow when I first heard this I didn't understand it very well, but as I grew up, little by little, this idea sank into my brain.

Now I can really say this is a great thought. LEARN SOMETHING NEW EVERY DAY. I'd add something to this thought: If I don't learn something new, I at least review what I have learned. I also discard what I don't need. This way I can have a lot of new ideas or at least go over older ideas.

All of my life I have built on this inner thought given to me by an early teacher. I do this with my writing. I do a little every day and think about what I am writing. I read it over, I try to find mistakes and give the ideas I wrote down much thought.

I say to myself, "Sam, you're eighty-two. What have you learned? Are you learning something new every day?" Little by little, I find myself getting better, particularly in my speciality, drumming. This is important to me because it helps to reinforce my mental concept of myself and my subject.

I do a great deal of writing about the drums, and I even learn something new from my own writings. What a wonderful thing that is . . . to learn from my own musical thoughts.

I try not to miss a day without learning something new. I'm writing this on July 4th, Independence Day. It's one of the biggest holidays of the year in this country. Some would think I'm nuts if I told them that I was in my studio writing. "It's a holiday," they would say. "Why are you working?"

Well, I'm not working. I am doing what I love. And I love what I do. To me, it's better than a good meal, better than a vacation. I write just enough to satisfy my love for writing and my need to put my thoughts on paper.

What did I learn today? I learned never to let a day slip by without learning something new.

Think

We all have a brain. As we get older, we begin to understand this machine that has been built into a most perfect design. This brain is where we have all of our information. When we wake up in the morning after some good sleep and rest, the brain is ready to go to work for us.

Each of us has a head that houses our brain. We have hair on our heads, two eyes, two ears to hear with, and then we have a nose that allows us to bring clear air into our heads that hold our brain. Our mouth allows the fuel to enter and nourish our bodies and our hearts as well as all the important parts of this entire unique system that allows us to function each day.

As we grow, we learn how to use our brain to think. Some of us become doctors, others accountants; some become teachers, others mechanics and build cars, planes, trains. Some of us learn music and others learn to be talk show hosts. Still others make recordings or films or videos, and some of us learn to program or use computers.

All of us, no matter what we do, must learn to use the brain to THINK. Thinking is what our brain is used for, and the better we can think, the better we can become in our chosen fields.

We can learn to think out our problems. We can create something that others can use or enjoy. Just think of this: our brain can help us to create a Broadway show or Hollywood movie, like TITANIC, CATS, A CHORUS LINE, or THE PRODUCERS. It can compose the music, the libretto of an opera, the orchestration of the music and how it must be played, costumes, lighting, and all of the parts that go together to make a stage show or a film. Just fantastic!

Special brains can think up so many special things: How to get a ROCKET TO THE MOON or TO MARS and then bring it back to earth. These are special people's brains. Just marvelous.

You who are reading this book can also THINK. All you have to do is think and then put your thinking to use. Simple, isn't it? Maybe not. But if you do enough of it you'll see that it gets easier every day as you develop your thinking processes. Who knows? You may come up with an important invention or maybe write a book about what you do and how you do it and why you'll continue to do what YOU LOVE TO DO IN YOUR LIFE.

THINK, THINK, THINK, THINK and never stop THINKING. It's great fun and can make your life exciting. My life is exciting — and I'm still thinking.

You Can Exercise in Many Places

"I don't have the time to exercise." "I don't have the time to go to a gym." "I really don't know how to exercise." "I'm so busy that I can't find the time to work out." Excuses, excuses.

That's all I hear from my friends and many other people, who say they can't fit a fitness program into their lives. Nonsense. Bull—. I always say, if you want to, you can do anything. There are twenty-four hours in a day and if you THINK, you'll see there is some time you can contribute to staying in good physical health and good shape. You'll find that staying in condition will give you great satisfaction, mostly because you feel good once you have done your daily workout. It's true even if you do only a part of that workout.

You can do it if you want to. Let me tell you what I do: the first thing I did was to get myself some free weights. I have ten-pounders, fifteen-pounders and twenty-pounders. I bought two sets of each. One set for my apartment and the other set to keep at my drum studio.

For five minutes in the morning, I lift the ten-pounders, fifteen-pounders and twenty-pounders. Some days I do ten minutes or fifteen minutes depending on where I have to be early in the morning. Then in the afternoon I do the same at my drum studio and then when I come home at night, I do another ten minutes. Simple as all that. I don't need to go to a gym to do my routines. I save dollars and don't waste time traveling to the gym. Exercising at home, I have time to take a bath and listen to my Yankees baseball team. Lots of free time. If I'm sitting on the "pot," I do a few lifts while on the "pot."

If I'm having breakfast at home, I have the weights at my feet and do a few lifts. If I'm watching TV, I do some more body conditioning. I have my weights on my bed and lift while I'm lying down.

There is always time to do a few more exercises. If I'm at my studio, waiting for a student, I do a few more sets of lifts. I do bend overs with the twenty-pounders, I lift them up to the ceiling with both hands. My students come and I stop, but during the day I do a good share of lifting and stretching. It makes my shoulders stronger every day. I try to keep my neck strong. I do three-quarter squats with the ten-pounders, then change to the fifteen-pounders and end the routine with the twenty-pounders.

There's always time in my day. You can do it too, once you set your mind to how it can be done.

Don't Tell People What You Are Going To Do . . . Do It!

"I'm going to cut a new CD." "I'm going to make a video." "I'm going to write a new book." On and on it goes. Don't brag about what you are going to do. I always say, do what you are going to do. Don't tell everybody what you might do, or where you are expecting to work. This is all talk. As they say, talk is cheap. MONEY TALKS, BS WALKS. Know what I mean?

If you like to hear yourself talk about the great things you are going to achieve and then never do them, that's dangerous. You may tell people you are working with this band or that band, and all of a sudden you notice no one calls you, and you wonder and can't understand why you are not working.

Well, you've told people you were so busy, they figured you are not available. So they got someone else.

This is a good lesson to learn. Keep your mouth shut. Over my many years in the music business I have found the less I told people of my expected accomplishments the better.

Do your "thing," complete it and then, when you have a finished product, you can show it or tell people about it. If a producer or record company asks you if you have a finished CD master and you want them to be interested in what you do and have done, the finished product will be sufficient. It will show the company or band leader who might like to use you and wants to hear how you sound and what you can do. The finished CD or photos or cassettes are good to have.

So many of us start things and never finish what we have started. Be a doer. Someone who gets things done. This gives you a chance to be a stronger person than someone who talks too much. "I'm going to this and that," and "I will be doing a concert as soon as I know the details." Talking or bragging because you want others to think you are busy can backfire on you.

When I was in my twenties, I did a lot of baloneying. Not good. Now, at eighty-two, my philosophy of life is to do my thing and complete it and if I need it, have it ready.

When I wrote *I Love What I Do!* I wrote it, had it edited, and my publishers had something that they felt could be an important book. That remains to be seen as things unfold. But my best advice is: **Do it. Don't talk about what you're going to do.** And about the old saying, "Talk is Cheap," it could cost you in the long run.

Do You Have a Hobby?

All of my life I have had hobbies. I saved stamps, I saved baseball cards, matchbook covers . . . I used to be interested in football and I would cut out all kinds of pictures of football players and glue them into a notebook. I covered the pictures with cellophane and wrote the player's name, the date, the team, and game that the news photo described. I had all kinds of hobbies and I always thought this was very healthy for me.

As I got older, I became more and more involved with my drumming. Eventually my music became the main thrust in my life. I loved it so much there wasn't a day I wouldn't study and practice for hours. I eventually realized this was making me a one-sided person.

I began to read more: newspapers and magazines and some books. I became more aware of the written word and this was a good change in my daily living.

One of my main hobbies, even now at eighty-two, is my interest in the New York Yankees. I found that team, like most teams, was very professional. I still get *Sporting News* and other baseball publications. I like to read about how ballplayers train.

Along with my baseball magazines, I read through physical fitness publications. This is because I keep up with my body conditioning routines. I know more than ever that staying in top shape is so important. Friends who didn't take care found as they grew older that their legs started to deteriorate. They have problems walking, bending, and doing the things we need our legs for. By lifting weights, I keep the upper and lower parts of my body in pretty good condition.

Frankly, I'm almost a fanatic about this. I have told myself: "SAM, YOU MUST TRAIN AND STAY IN TIP-TOP SHAPE IF YOU WISH TO BE ABLE

TO BE ACTIVE TOMORROW AND THE NEXT DAY AND THE DAY AFTER THAT."

So, over the years, a number of very practical things have become both my hobbies and a part of my life. It's great at my age to be able to see this as being important. And it is. Make no bones about it. If you don't know this, as I said in my earlier book, YOU'LL PAY THE PRICE EVEN IF YOU DON'T PAY THE PRICE.

I think we all should have hobbies. Play chess for the mind, or a card game once in a while. Listen to music, collect recordings of all kinds of music: Jazz, Latin, Broadway, etc. Keep your hobbies up. Don't let them get away from you.

You don't need to devote many hours a day to this form of fun. Perhaps a half-hour or an hour . . . WHATEVER YOU CAN CONTRIBUTE TO THINGS THAT YOU WOLD LOVE TO BE INVOLVED WITH.   That should help satisfy your desires. It does mine. And the more I think of this, the greater the pleasure I get from it.

GET A HOBBY. GET A FEW HOBBIES. This is healthy for your brain and your life.

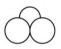

What Do You Think You Will Leave After You're Gone?

While it may be early for some to think of this subject, I've given a lot of thought as to what will happen to all of the materials I will be leaving to others, as the song says, AFTER I'M GONE. It's something that all of us should give some deep thought to. What will happen to our life's work? How will it go on in the future? We can't know, but while we are still healthy and able, we should think about what we would like to happen to what we leave behind.

I have a few thousand books, videos, audio tapes, and magazines that I have produced. The instruction materials for drummers was a major part of my life, because I am so involved in the music world. I'm involved in performing, education, and most of the creative parts in my field. I would like to think that my work will go on.

So I must put down on paper what I want to happen to this wide collection of material that I have developed. I think we all have to spell it out, because only we can know what we want to happen to a lifetime of work. If we are one of those who create, we should put pen to paper, listing what should happen to the material we developed.

I have been writing down, little by little, what I want to happen to the vast body of information I have documented. I am thinking a great deal about this and about how I can put this material into hands that will keep it alive, long after I have passed through this world.

Many of us have no idea as to what we want done with our "left-overs," as I call them. What to do? That is the question.

We can leave our things to our family. But in my case, would my family know what to do with drum material? No one else in my family has ever played the drums. No one has an inkling about what I do. How can they, when, as in all busy families, everyone fends for themselves and so are not involved with the rest of the family.

So the question now for each of us is: **WHAT DO WE WANT DONE WITH WHAT WE LEAVE BEHIND WHEN WE LEAVE THIS EARTH?** Interesting, isn't it? For me, at age eighty-two, not knowing how long I will be on earth motivates me to think about the future of my work.

I suggest you give this some serious thought. Seek a lawyer who knows about wills and how to handle all of your important contributions to the world so that they will go on after you. Talk to people who know and may be able to direct you. Sit down and write out what you are leaving behind, what is important about it, and what should be done with your ideas and contributions.

Get some answers and hope it is what you want done with everything. For myself, I think I am coming up with ideas that I would like to see put into effect. **TIME WILL TELL.**

What Are Your Thoughts About Love?

Good topic! How do you feel about love? Where does it fit into your life? How important is it to each of us? Have you given it much thought? Have you ever been in love? What does that mean to you? Have you been able to put love into your life while trying to maintain a professional career?

So many questions we need to answer . . . and we will all answer differently. That's what makes it interesting to me.

For myself, I have experienced great love, beautiful love and, like all of us, some disappointments in love. Love can get very complicated and many times disrupt our lives. Love can make us satisfied with living and make us do great things. Then again, some not great things. We sometimes can do foolish things when we think we are in love. The most interesting part of all of this is, how do we handle love when it comes to us?

When we are in love, we never know why we are in love. We sometimes can't explain the wonderful feeling we get when we fall in love. However, I always tell people that they can't let love disrupt their professional lives.

There are many parts to being in love: The great SEX THAT MIGHT DEVELOP BETWEEN YOU AND THE ONE YOU LOVE, the wonderful feeling of being with someone who loves you, and your feeling of love for them. As the song says, "LOVE IS A MANY SPLENDORED THING." And it is — I think.

In my eighty-two years, I've been in love a few times. When I got married, I thought I was in love. I was twenty-six when I got married. I never really knew anything about love. I thought I did, of course, but I didn't know beans about it. In fact, I never knew why I got married. I got married because that was what I thought I was supposed to do as a young fellow. May I say at this time, I was so wrong. I never understood what was going on with my life.

I realized I was married to my drums but that was okay because it was a tremendous learning experience. I've never regretted it. I learned fast. Since I was a good student I knew how to learn, take direction, and get educated. Marriage was an education for me. Developing my brain and my body and understanding love better was all so good for me.

By the way, I am still learning about the other half of life, about myself and women. I'm certain that we all learn as we get older and grow.

To me, being loved and loving someone is so important and great for all of us. Now that I am reaching eighty-three, I know a little more about love and what I did wrong in my early involvement with love. We can't learn it from a book, we must live it and experience it. Once you have, you will really know when love comes along.

Are You a Gambler in Life?

Don't get me wrong when I pose the question: are you a gambler in life? I do not mean in cards, dice, or horses, or even betting on a football game, a boxing match, or Lotto.

No. I am not talking about that form of gambling. By the way, if you are a habitual gambler, I suggest you seek help from Gambler's Anonymous. That organization can help you. However, you must first want to help yourself and then they can help you.

The kind of gambling I'm talking about is when you take chances in your life; where you do things and take that chance that you can have things work for you or against you. I am a gambler on my talents. I do things that I feel will work for me. I have never invested in the stock market, where someone else is handling my dollars. I invest in my talents and feel I can be successful when I do my thing.

When I write a new book, I pay my dollars to publish it. I feel that there are enough people in my industry who like what I do to make me almost ninety-five-percent sure that my new book will be successful. I must like what I write and publish and give my material a chance to succeed. Many times it has. Yes, I have some books that have bombed out. I expect that. But at least I take my chances and invest my dollars in myself. I win some and sometimes I lose. However, I control my winning or losing. No one else invests my dollars for me. I want to control my own money and my chances.

If you have confidence in yourself and your abilities and there are things you wish to do in your life, I say, **GO FOR IT**. Try your best. At least you'll know that you've tried and didn't wait or depend on others.

I have musician friends who look for a record company to produce their records. You write a song and someone else owns the copyright. You write a film or show and have others produce it and then others own part of what you have produced. You might get very little return while others reap the harvest and you may become very unhappy because you gave your soul away.

When I write a book or create something it becomes like one of my children. I wouldn't want to sell my children. My creations are all mine. Good, bad, or otherwise, I want to own all my innovations and ideas. I own them and no one else. My first book and second book I own. It's being published by nice people, but the copyright is mine. And that's how I like it!

Crazy as it seems, this is important to me. As I've said, I am a gambler in my life. I do take chances when I create and publish or develop my ideas. If I am successful, good for me. If I blow it, so be it. That is how it is. Que Sera, Sera. ("What Will Be, Will Be," as the song says.)

Are You Certain That You Will Reach Your Goals?

Nothing in this life is certain. Nothing in this world is guaranteed. We don't come into this world with papers saying that what we do is going to be the way we want it. I have learned a lot in my eighty-two years and now I know that the only way for Sam Ulano to get ahead was to break my butt and work myself to the bone. Maybe then and only then would I reach my goals.

Somewhere I've read that nothing comes easy. Nothing in life is as simple as we might think it is. I don't know if people out there reading this philosophy of my life think everything is a snap. You snap your fingers and bango(!), your goals are reached and you have achieved what you set your mind to do.

Like the story says, we live it out and there is a beginning and there is an end. Sometimes we don't know the ending because we are not alive for the final part of the story. That makes sense to me.

In fact, the other day I was discussing with one of my students what she is after in her life and what she was doing to reach her goals. She said she keeps studying hard every day and practices her instruments every day. Little by little, she says, she can see her goals being reached. LITTLE BY LITTLE. (By the way, she is a professional harpist and studies drums so she can have a better understanding of the reading of rhythm, the breakdown of the value of notes, and how to count and play the various notations.) It's an interesting study. She knows there's a great deal more to go, but she is on the right track and can see the light at the end of the tunnel.

We all should have goals and try to develop a system for a way to reach the plateaus we set for ourselves. I have set my goals over the years and then day by day I try to find the best method to reach them. I do this for myself every day. Many times I reach my goals. I make sure I don't set the levels too high so that I don't shoot too high and make my goals unattainable. I take my goals each at a special pace and STICK WITHIN MY BOUNDARIES.

I've had many goals. I've worked hard to accomplish each goal, and when I do I feel it helps me succeed in my profession and live my life without cutting myself off. Setting expectations that are too high can be dangerous. Make things simple for yourself. This way you can reach your goals.

The More I Think About It, the More I Realize the Importance of Our Legs

I've written about our legs in *I Love What I Do!* Once again I stress the point. Whenever I ride a bus here in New York City and see someone in a wheelchair, I thank my lucky stars that my legs are still strong and can still get me where I wish to go.

If your legs are gone, someone has to help you get around. If your legs are damaged and out of commission, you will have a problem. For myself, as I wrote, my legs are a very important part of playing my drums. I have two pedals. One is used with the right foot and one with the left. When my legs are gone, that will be the end of my ability to perform. Then there's getting to the place of the performance; carrying my drums, transporting them from my home to the place where I will have to play. And back again!

The reason I once again tell you about taking care of your legs and sticking to it is because without the use of our legs we just can't operate our bodies. I learned this lesson many years ago and I drilled it into my subconscious mind. "Don't forget to exercise your legs, Sam," I would tell myself. "Keep them strong." From my thighs down to my toes, I exercise each and every day.

When I wake up in the morning, before I get out of bed, I stretch my legs from a prone position. I raise each leg up one hundred times. First the right leg, then one hundred stretches with the left. I say to myself, "Never let it go, Sam. Never let it go."

I bring my legs up to my waist and stretch them back to the flat position on my bed. I turn and let my legs hang off of the bed. I lift up from the floor and back again down to the floor. One hundred times. Each leg. Each morning.

Each morning, before I leave my apartment, I stand up and do short squats, almost a three-quarter squat. I never go all the way down because I do not want to strain my knees. This is a great exercise. Every day, about one hundred squats. Only three quarters of the way down; never missing a day.

I feel that I can't impress upon you enough that you should start taking care of your legs early. This will make your entire body feel so good. I sometimes do this three-quarter squat with my crossbar. It's about a sixty-pound bar and I do one hundred squats one hundred times. I do this at my practice studio where I keep the sixty-pound crossbar on an adjustable crossbar. When I say "adjustable crossbar," I am talking about a bar that I can either add or take off weight. **Do it every day**. You'll enjoy the results. You'll be happy with them. I know I am!

Do You Like Yourself?

I remember, some years ago, my dear friend and the world's greatest drummer, MR. BUDDY RICH, and I were having a conversation with a number of other famous drummers backstage at the famed jazz club, THE BOTTOM LINE (at 4th Street and Mercer, here in Manhattan). The discussion was about whether he, Buddy Rich, liked himself. Buddy said, "If I didn't like me, no one else would." He was saying that he felt he didn't care if others liked him, he had to like himself first.

Of course, this was quite a few years ago, and, now that I have digested this idea, I find it's so true. I've come to the same conclusion. YES, I LIKE ME. In fact, I LOVE ME. This is why I LOVE WHAT I DO. It really has been the important part of why I love what I do and it all fits together.

I've found that if I liked myself, others would like me too. Whether they did or not was not the most important part of my life, but it is good to have others like you. I've heard others say they can't stand themselves and wish they were someone else. Unfortunately, we can't be someone else. We are who we are.

I think it's nice to love yourself. To like yourself means to me that you are a nice person. Someone once said, it's nice to be a person but it's nicer to be a nice person. This is so true. If I like me, I can stand myself. I find it easier to understand my faults. We all have faults and we all have to understand these faults and live with ourselves, faults and all. Accept your faults and maybe you just may wind up liking yourself!

So, what do I like about myself? I hope this doesn't sound too conceited to you, because I don't mean it that way. I don't want to sound like I'm bragging. What do I like about myself? I like my talent and I like what I can do with my talents. I like the satisfaction of what I do in my field and feel that I am contributing to the music world. The feeling that I am creating and adding to my field gives me a sort of inner satisfaction.

Even writing this book, I feel that I am revealing things about myself that makes me happy. I feel that I am not selfish about my work and wish to spread the word so that someone reading this might gain from my inner thoughts.

I must say that I feel I am completely happy with my life, what I am, and who I am. Some people never find themselves, never find what they love in life and go through a daily struggle trying to find themselves. It's too bad, because if you know who you are, you might do many things with your life. I can honestly say to you, I like me and what I'm about.

Do You Believe There Is a Strong Power Watching Over You? Maybe Motivating You?

Have you ever given this some thought? Do you think there is a strong outside power that is watching over you and giving you the strength to do what you do? Do you think that this outside force is part of your existence and gives you the inner self force to start and complete, create, and develop yourself so that you feel you can go on and reach the highest peak?

Does this sound crazy to you? Because I must confess that I have felt for many years, almost back to when I was ten or so, that something, some powerful feeling was in me and this great strength was what made and makes **Sam Ulano tick**. The only way I can define this to you is that this ever exciting force is so embedded inside my body and mind that I can't help feel that it is what makes me do what I do. I feel it's a gift that some special force is part of my life. Where does this power come from? I don't know but I feel it every day.

Some nights I go to sleep feeling like I am on the wrong track. In the morning, the feeling I had when I went to sleep, that empty feeling, is gone and I have this renewed feeling that what I was doing will all work out. Now I can't explain feeling one way the night before and waking up and feeling everything is all right again.

Then I go through my paces. I take medication in the morning, take my bath, get dressed nicely, and head to my studio, where I teach and write. I am full of excitement facing the new day. It's really incredible and fills me with wondering about the future. I am curious how the day will end up.

Yesterday is gone. I did whatever I was able to do with the twenty-four hours of the day that I had. Now, today I have a new twenty-four hours to work with.

Yes, I do believe there is a stronger power that makes me do what I am doing. Some days, working on my philosophy book, I can do just a page or two. Sometimes nothing. But I can always do a page or at least think of something I want to add to the book. Today it's July 6th, a Friday, and it's about 11:30 in the morning. I have done nine full pages, one after another and I'm still writing. It's just insane how this works. I'm a half-baked typist. I make lots of mistakes but I can get my ideas down on paper — and I'm still going.

Where does this energy come from? Why does it happen this way? How can the brain create as it does? It's remarkable and thrills me that I can do this.

Are You Envious of Others?

I have been lucky all of these years: I honestly never was ENVIOUS OF OTHER PEOPLE IN MY FIELD OR IN OTHER FIELDS.

I've always been happy for people who are successful in their lives. I have never felt, "Why doesn't that happen to me? I think I'm better than so and so." These kinds of thoughts never entered my mind. I guess it's because I have been so busy with my own life, I've never had the time to sit and brood that the other fellow was getting all the glory.

I really learned a great deal from those who were on top. Listening and watching them was an education for me. I like to see success, because I appreciate the hard work it takes for someone to reach that high level of recognition. Whatever they gained from their hard work, I have always felt they deserved.

If you feel sorry for yourself or concentrate on what others are reaping from their great abilities, then you might have problems reaching your goals. As you get older, this is a lesson you should learn. Being envious of your colleagues in your work gets you nothing and many times can be dangerous for you. Allow others to have their day in the sun. When you grow to be that skilled and become recognized in your field, your turn will come.

Tony Martin once said that he never wanted to be top dog. He just wanted to be good enough so those who liked what he did would pay attention to him. Fighting others because you are not getting your piece of the pie is not a good way to be.

I've never gone to hear another drummer and sat in the audience saying to myself that I could play better than the fellow on stage. Or asking myself, why aren't I the drummer? I learn from watching and listening to what other players are doing.

Envy can make you angry at the world. It's sort of like feeling the parade is passing you by. Do your own thing. Develop your talents. Try your best to reach your goals.

I have been playing for many years now and have taught many top people in the percussion field. Many of my students have become teachers, and many have played in all phases of the music world. I am so happy for them, and I teach with the desire that my pupils make the best of their talents.

I don't envy my students. It never enters my thoughts. I couldn't do what I do if this envy was inside my mind, my heart, my guts. No way would I allow this to happen to me.

You should examine your inner feelings. If you find yourself envious of people who do what you do, stop it now as you search your heart. Make sure this trait is not a part of your makeup. **No, I never have been or will be envious of another's success. More power to them.**

Do You Study Yourself Day After Day?

Think about this: Every day we get a new chance to improve ourselves. If you have a day in which things aren't working out for you, keep in mind that it's not the end of the world. The very next day you can work on what didn't go right for you and correct what wasn't the way you wanted it to be. I have learned this lesson well. Next year I will be eighty-three, and I see myself having another year where I can improve myself.

If I've made a lot of mistakes this year, I make sure that I will not repeat the same mistakes next year. Every day is a chance to try to find better ways to handle my money, to improve my writing, my drumming, how to stay on top of my body conditioning. There are many things that I have improved each year. Day by day I work at keeping my system going, while working on adding to my ideas and staying on top of my game.

When I was younger, I was in a hurry to get things done. Not a good idea. Gradually I began to pace myself and give much thought to how I was living my life. Today I stick with the three things that are most important to me: MY HEALTH, MY EDUCATION, AND MY FINANCES.

Taking care of my health first means that I will be in good condition to develop my education, not only in playing my drums, but in many phases of my education. And that includes trying to speak better and trying to stay dressed properly.

SOME GROWN-UPS DRESS SLOPPILY!

Some adults have said to me it's their way of communicating with their kids. Nonsense. The young must learn from adults. We teach them. They eventually mature and are able to teach their children or the youngsters they will meet.

Finally, taking care of my dollars to make sure I have enough to pay my rent and living expenses is very important. Throughout *I LOVE WHAT I DO!* and here again, I stress these three points of my life. I think eventually you will come to the same conclusions that I have.

As I move along with my life I always come back to the fact that I can always improve myself the next day. At this point, I am very happy with my life. I feel good and don't have to overeat and get fat again. I am content with where I am at eighty-two; however, I want to be able to approach ninety in the best shape I can.

I have set up a mental concept for myself that as I get older I want to be able to walk and do all the things that my legs can now do. I want to have my diabetes under the best control that I can; keep my weight down; take my medication and listen to my doctors at the VETERANS HOSPITAL. They watch me like a hawk. I take regular blood tests and keep my medication under observation at all times. I study myself day by day and make sure I'm where I want to be with my life. It's a lesson I have learned very well. Think about that. Check yourself every day.

Remember, the World Doesn't Owe You Anything

The lyric of a famous song, "I'VE GOT THE WORLD ON A STRING" says a great deal. Many people think that the world owes them a living and that they don't have to work to get better. They think that they can just sit back and everything will come to them. What a crock of nonsense. Each of us must make our way and try our best so we can earn the rewards we get for the effort we put into being the best we can. When we reach some of our goals, we can get back some of the bucks we paid to study and get paid for the many hours, days, and years of our lives we put into getting better.

Many times I hear people bitching about how much doctors charge. No one remembers that doctors went without a lot when they studied. They gave up many of the enjoyments in life to study hard in order to become a good doctor.

Many years of study and practice go into becoming a top-notch professional musician. When musicians go out to play at night, others dance to the music. People are enjoying themselves because each day of their lives these professional musicians practice, train, and learn their craft so they can go out at night to play for the enjoyment of the dancing and dining public.

I have spent many years and countless hours learning my drums. I can play now and get back some of the dollars I previously invested so I can live a life where I can afford my daily existence. I spend hours giving others drum lessons so they can play as professionals. I give the students a career, and they now can be part of the music world. Many of my students are some of the better drummers. These young students became adults and now make a good income.

Thus, anyone who thinks everything is coming to them gratis has another thing coming. I am certain as you grow up and mature you begin to understand that nothing comes easily. The world doesn't owe you a thing.

I believe you get out of something what you put into it. In fact, if you put a lot into the pot, you may even take out more than just a fair share. I have worked at studying and busting my tail and now at the age of eighty-two, I'm getting a great deal out of the pot. When I say you may get more than you contributed, I really think this is true. I see it with myself.

People in my profession are always giving me back so much in pleasure and success. It's a marvelous feeling as my days unfold. Don't expect someone to bring you success on a silver platter. "As you sow, so shall you reap," (or something like that). That's what the Bible says. **It's true!**

Who Motivates You?

This interests me. I try every day to find who motivates me, and, as I investigate this question, I come up with all kinds of answers. However, I never was able to put my finger on THE answer. WHO MOTIVATES SAM ULANO?

I get all kinds of thoughts about it, and then, just when I have an idea as to what sets me off, bingo, it's not what I thought. I then look for another answer. However, you know what? I've decided it really isn't that important as to what makes this happen.

Just the other day my brother Ben and I were talking about my first book. Ben asked, "What made you write it? What came over you that made you want to put your ideas down on paper?" I said, "Ben, I really can't say what it was and why and how my mind and computer brain started to write. But before I knew it I had written twenty pages and my hands just kept typing. Then before I knew it, I had fifty-four pages done and I thought I needed it edited."

I found Ed Petoniak's name in a XEROX SHOP. I jotted it down and although I didn't know him from a hole in the wall, I gave him a call. We started to become friends and I paid him to edit for me. He began bringing me sections of the material I gave him, edited and set up on a computer disk.

Then, as we finished editing the first fifty-four pages, I found I had more to add, and the next thing you know, I had ninety-two pages! One thing led to another and the next thing I know I had made contact with David Richard, the Publishing Director of Vital Health Publishing/ENHANCEMENT BOOKS. He felt I had written something worth publishing. He asked me how I felt about his company publishing *I LOVE WHAT I DO!* We talked about and discussed a contract, and before you know it, the book was ready.

I told my brother Ben that it was like someone who writes a hit song and doesn't know the song is a hit. Before one knows it, like a fairy tale, the hit song becomes number one in the world and there it is. Go explain it. I can't.

It's a beautiful ride in life, because I honestly don't know how or why these great things in our lives happen. **WHO MOTIVATES ME?** I'm a big believer in **GOD**. I can't prove it, but I think **GOD** is watching over people like us and gives us the inspiration to do things with our brains and bodies. Does this sound silly or strange to you?

Here I sit at my **BROTHER TYPEWRITER** (that's the name of the company), with my **HUNT** and **PECK** system; one finger at a time . . . well, actually, two fingers at a time . . . (one finger on each hand). I pour out my thoughts. And so I said to my brother, I can't explain it. That's just how it is.

Who knows? I might even come up with enough material for a third book. It could happen.

Do You Believe in God?

Many times I have been asked this question — DO YOU BELIEVE IN GOD? — and, if so, what makes you have this feeling? I can't explain it but for many years I have had this inner belief that something or someone was watching over me. All my life I would tell people I know that I was a very lucky person because a certain power or spirit was taking care of me.

When I was in the Army, during World War Two, and I left home and family and was traveling to Kentucky, Alabama, then across the Pacific Ocean to HAWAII and near the end of the war was living in Japan with the occupational forces, all this time, I never worried because this feeling inside of me that GOD, whatever and wherever God is, was looking after me.

I have had this feeling even very recently. As I was approaching my eighty-second birthday, I would wake up every morning and say, THANK YOU GOD. Here is another great day that I could do some more writing, practice my drums and advance in what I love to do. These days it is even stronger. I can't tell you why I feel this way but it stays with me everywhere I go.

I am certain I'm not the only person who feels this way. I ask myself sometimes, why did I write book one of my philosophy of life at eighty and then start writing a second book about living life and doing the things I do. When I play with a band, I get a feeling that I can keep drumming for many years. The excitement of being on the band stand and leading my group of musicians — what a charge I get! Some people lose their desire for things in life, yet with me, I am so inspired to feel I still can perform and enjoy my musical life more each day.

I have this strong inner glow that never seems to die out. When I go to sleep at night I look up and out my window and thank my lucky stars that GOD IS DIRECTING ME ALL THE TIME. I have never

lost my belief in the power of this feeling. I have never felt that
GOD has stopped caring and watching over me. Like the song
says, SOMEONE TO WATCH OVER ME. Yes, I do believe in GOD, or
what I call GOD. I feel we all have to believe in something. My
brain and mind say THAT MY GOD OR THIS POWER IS IN ME. I think
it's in all of us, but I don't know if each of us has recognized
HIM/HER or whatever form GOD takes in our minds. I'm Jewish,
so I'd guess my GOD IS JEWISH.

For me, I have GOD IN MY HEART, AND I'M CERTAIN HE HAS BEEN
TAKING CARE OF ME AND MY LIFE AND WHAT I DO.

That's the best I can tell you for now.

Do You Know Where You Are Heading?

I have asked this question of myself over these many years: Do I really know where I am going in my life? I have always said it would be a good idea if I had a direction to go with my life. It's a good question and I pose it here for you. DO YOU, WHO ARE READING THIS, HAVE AN IDEA WHERE YOU ARE GOING IN YOUR LIFE and WHAT DO YOU WANT OUT OF YOUR LIFE? Do you wake up in the morning with an idea of WHAT YOU WANT TO BE AS YOU GROW OLDER?

Do you think you'll reach eighty-two, looking forward to eighty-three as I am? Do you expect in your life to reach eighty-two? Do you look forward to accomplishing your life's dreams? Will you reach your goals? Interesting, isn't it?

I never gave it much thought, but I did have a feeling that Sam Ulano would reach eighty and would go on to reach ninety and maybe a lot more. I set out my plan that if I take good care of the body that was entrusted to me, if I am careful and don't expect too much from myself, I just might get to ninety years of age.

When I get to ninety, I will make plans to reach one hundred and be in the best shape I can be. I still expect to be very active; teaching some more drummers; writing a few more of my drum instruction books; doing my exercises and lifting weights on a daily basis. I plan to eat properly, take my diabetes medication, and listen to the doctors who have taken care of me all of these years. I know I might just reach my goals.

I might even write a few more books as to how I see life at the ripe old age of one hundred! I expect to continue to play skillful professional drums because I am a skilled percussion man, not just because I'm elderly. In my mind I expect to be a young old man, a man at one hundred who thinks with a young mind. I know it can be done and in my "computer brain," I have set these thoughts in motion.

So I ask you out there, **DO YOU KNOW WHERE YOU ARE HEADING?** Will you get all the things done in your life that **YOU SET OUT TO DO?** Will you find the happiness that makes life worth living? Will you have the strength to do at eighty what you could do at sixty? How does this look to you at the age you are now, reading this philosophy of mine?

Has anybody asked you these questions? Have you made plans to complete your dreams and goals? I'll tell you this: It's not easy. No one said it would be. I think it's easy if you are in good health, if your mind isn't mixed up from the problems of day-to-day living. It takes a strong will and perseverance to forge ahead. Take it from me. When I wake up I set my **MIND CLOCK TO KEEP MY BODY TICKING.** With my feeling for **GOD** and His help keeping me thinking straight, I think I can do it . . . **SO CAN YOU.**

My Thoughts on Smoking and Drinking

Someone asked me, at my age, what have I learned about these vices? How do I feel about them? Do I think I would have liked being involved with any of these parts of life?

To tell you the truth, I can't really speak as an expert on this subject. I did smoke, but I never considered myself a real smoker. I was up to two or three packs of cigarettes a day. But now that I can reflect back on my experience with smoking, I can honestly say I never really enjoyed smoking. I sort of did it because I thought it was a "hip" thing to do.

As I have followed many of the reports about tobacco and what it does to our bodies, I really can say I am happy that I gave it up many years ago. I haven't had a cigarette in my mouth for so many years now that it is never on my mind. In fact, I have no recollection of what smoking was like. Now, with the reports that have come out saying that smoking is dangerous to your health, that it causes cancer and does other terrible things to our bodies, I don't regret giving it up.

In today's times, a pack costs around seven dollars and in some places more. I am really glad I have given the habit up. I feel sorry for those who are hooked on smoking. **SEVEN DOLLARS A DAY. WOW, THAT'S A LOT OF MONEY FOR JUST A PACK.** If you smoke two or three packs a day, you are spending a lot of money each day and also doing a great deal of damage to your body.

I gave it up "cold turkey." I just stopped and never bought a pack again. I haven't had matches in my house or in my pockets since then. I can't stand being around people who are smoking. I almost can say **I HATE IT.** I don't tell others to stop smoking, I just avoid people who puff all day on smokes. I can't stand the odor that comes from a smoker's mouth. It is horrible. Not my cup of tea.

Man, I can't stand being near people who smoke or drink. When those two habits are combined, it's terrible. Even social drinking at parties, weddings, or nightclubs is one of the most distasteful things to me. I can't stand it and don't want to be around those who think it's "hep" to drink and get "bombed." Just not good. If you are someone who drinks, I feel sorry for you. You numb your brain; you can't drive; and in the long run you do serious damage to your body.

The human body wasn't meant to be abused with liquor. If that's what you like, so be it. But I don't need it, don't like it, and don't wish to be part of this phase of life. **DRINKING. OUCH!**

As for **DRUGS**, well you don't need Sam Ulano to tell you what a horrible thing this is. I never experimented with drugs. I have never been drunk or "high" and don't care to even have the thought enter my mind.

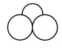

How Do You Handle Holidays?

O nce I heard someone say that holidays are the loneliest days of the year. I don't know, because I love all holidays. I never had the feeling of loneliness. I guess I am fortunate because I have something to fill my days. I am eighty-two and I never remember being alone and feeling sad when the holidays came.

I love New Year's Eve, because I have always played with my band at some special affair. I play my drums and meet so many nice people I can talk to that night. I never had to spend money somewhere because I wasn't working and found I had to go out to enjoy myself.

Then I have fun at Christmas. I still believe in Santa Claus, and I like the presents I can give others and sometimes get. Just great fun and I love it. As for Thanksgiving . . . Well, here many times I have gone to someone's house for dinner — turkey and all the trimmings. A wonderful holiday.

I am fortunate not to have to be by myself. And if I am by myself, I am able to occupy my time. I write, practice, and sometimes play somewhere with my band. Again, I think back to what my mom said to my brothers and six sisters. My mom told everyone in my family that I was able to be by myself and enjoy my own company. Many of us have nothing to do and this means that we have to find a way to make the days fun.

I know the ability to enjoy these kind of days is not easy. I have known and still know friends of mine who feel that spending holidays with others is a problem. I can do so much or just loll around my house and I won't get the "blues," because I don't have to be with someone.

Of course, if you have someone you love and can enjoy their company, that's beautiful. If you are surrounded by family and they cook and invite you to spend the holidays with them, that's also wonderful. However, if you are someone who has learned how to be satisfied with your own company, that's also great.

It's wonderful if you have a way to occupy your holidays but, if not, that's something each of us has to deal with. I don't feel sorry for myself. I don't spend time thinking about this problem. I like myself and so I can be with myself all day or any amount of time. I HAVE NO PROBLEM WITH THIS. And I say, in all honesty, I can be by myself and not worry about it or I can spend time with friends, or family.

I know this about myself: I never needed others to fill my days. Either way, with someone or alone, I am in good shape when the holidays come upon us . . . Easter, Passover, St. Patrick's Day, the major Jewish holidays, Labor Day, the Fourth of July . . . you name it. I, Sam Ulano, can handle these days and enjoy myself when they come along.

These Ideas Are All My Own

The ideas in both of my Philosophy books are all my own. No one else influenced me in writing my Philosophy of Life. I put this together by myself. I never asked anyone to help me think this material out. I do think I'm adult enough to be able to write my thoughts down without someone else giving me advice as to what to write. I sat down at my typewriter and just decided to put down my concept of this book all on my own.

I am having fun going back in my life, reviewing what I did as I grew up and what I was and still am thinking about. At eighty-two, I have a great many ideas that make up each topic in the book.

I just type free-style, as if I'm talking to the reader. I just let my mind be free and say what I want to say. I try to describe the way things happened to me when I was younger and as I was growing. It comes so easy to me. I really don't know why but ideas just flow from my mind to my fingers as I type this book of my life.

I don't hold back and I don't try to make up stories. I tell it like it is. I've been asked by a few people, what made me want to write these books of mine? Good question. I heard someone once say we all have a book in our minds. Some of us put it on paper and others never do. Why, I can't say, but I feel that's how it is.

I'll go along with my drumming and all of a sudden a new idea for a new percussion book appears in my brain. I say, "Yeah, Sam, that's interesting. Why don't you write it? See how it looks and maybe the concept might be something important." There, once again, original ideas pop up in my brain.

I can honestly say I have read very little about other philosophies of life. I know there must be tons of material written about this phase of our lives. I know that others have put their ideas down on paper but others don't take the time to write.

Do we need to be inspired? Do we need to say to ourselves that if we write a book, maybe we'll make some money; get recognition; become famous; even make the best-seller list? Is this why we write about our talents, what we have accomplished? I don't know about others, but I never gave any of those things a second thought. I am having fun putting down what is going on in my mind. To me, it's thrilling.

It's so different from what I have been trained to do. My entire life I've been searching for ideas about drumming and discovering where these fit in with my life. Now I find I want to write these thoughts about my inner life and desires. Just fascinating.

How I Changed My Life

At the age of six I was told by my family that I had a boy soprano voice and would sing in Hebrew School. I had fun doing that and I never was concerned if I was special at singing. Then, as I got older, at about age thirteen, my voice changed and I stopped singing in Hebrew School. I just didn't do it any longer. My friend who lived in the same building, Harry Koppelman, bought a set of drums. They were new drums and I would be up in his apartment and bang on the drums. Harry started to take lessons and I soon joined him. We took a lesson a week from a gentleman who lived on the ground floor of our building. Harry paid him thirty-five cents a lesson and since Harry and I were very close pals, I joined him and also studied drums for thirty-five cents a lesson.

Jules Wishick had us buy a book called *The Harry Bower System*, and we started learning drums from this piece of literature. It was a nice chance for the two of us to pal around and have things to talk about.

At that time in my life, I was always out in the street playing what we called **STICK BALL**. We took the handle of a broom and had a **SPALDING BALL** and were part of a team on **SIMPSON STREET**. We played almost seven days a week.

I played the outfield. I wasn't too good, but like all youngsters I had so much pleasure from chasing the ball and trying to hit it. It was great exercise and wonderful to be a part of a team. However, one day, when I started studying the drums, I was out in the outfield and asked myself: **"SAM, HOW WILL YOU GET BETTER AT DRUMMING CHASING A BALL?"** Being outside I never practiced the drums and it came to me that I had to practice and study my notes. I walked off the field as if I was hypnotized . . . in a daze.

"I have to practice," I told the fellows on the field, and I went home to my apartment and started to practice drums six to eight hours every day. I even became a better student in school because I had to learn to be a better reader. Math played a big part in learning music and as I mentioned earlier, my math was awful. So I practiced and I studied hard.

This is how I changed my life. I had an inner feeling that I could be a good drum player. I really thought I could get the hang of playing my drums.

At that time, my brother, Al, saw something in me. He felt I had drum talent and he told me if I studied hard in school and at the drums, he would buy me my first set of drums. This was, as they say, an offer I couldn't refuse. This changed my life and my thinking. Before this time in my life, I really wasn't thinking of anything special. However, I was fascinated by the sound of drums and the idea of playing drums with a band.

BINGO. I got it. This was what I found I loved and wanted to learn how to do.

If at First You Don't Succeed,
Then You Only Have Yourself To Blame

I've borrowed the famous statement: If at first you don't succeed, try, try again. I've changed it a bit: IF AT FIRST YOU DON'T SUCCEED, THEN YOU ONLY HAVE YOURSELF TO BLAME. I like the way that sounds rather than the first version.

We must take some of the blame if things don't work out as we want them to work out. If you agree with my concept regarding how this famous slogan goes, then you realize that you have to WORK HARDER TO REALLY LEARN WHAT YOU WISH TO DO AND TO GET BETTER AT IT. YOU MUST PUT IN SPECIAL EFFORT AND STICK TO WHAT YOU WANT TO DO UNTIL YOU HAVE IT UNDER CONTROL.

Make sure you allow yourself time to think out what you wish to do and do some work each day until you see your ideas happening as you planned them. We never can succeed in a hurry. Take your time and you will get the results you seek. That's how I see it. Many an idea was not thought out. Many an idea didn't work out at first. However, with time you will put all the pieces in place and complete what you were trying to do.

In my field, I practice and practice, then I do it all over again, and wonder of wonders, I work out my problems and accomplish my goals. I tell you, it's marvelous how this happens. I give myself plenty of time and don't expect too much of myself. TRY, TRY AGAIN. I always come back to the original beginning and try to succeed without ever expecting it at first.

If it doesn't work out, I blame myself and tell myself that I must give it another shot. Sometimes I set my ideas aside for a week or a month or sometimes a couple of years. There are times I gave my ideas the best shot, and these ideas didn't work out as I thought they would. However, sometimes in the future, the idea comes back to me, and it all begins to make sense, and I find myself coming up with the answers I need.

I discovered as I grew older and understood what I was doing much better, that the experience of listening, learning, and taking direction from someone who could explain what I needed to know was crucial in having everything develop as I wanted. As you live your life from day to day, things look different than when you first started out. You can say to yourself, "I know what I'm doing." Again, as SY OLIVER, the famous arranger and composer always said: "IT'S SO EASY WHEN YOU KNOW HOW."

So, if at first you don't succeed, try it again and again and again. You'll get it. I know because it came to me and I did get it. Never think it can't be done. It can always be done.

Think Twice Before You Have Many Different Credit Cards

When I was twenty-six and newly married, I was very much engrossed in my development as a drummer and as a human being. I opened my drum studio a month after I was discharged from the U.S. ARMY BAND. I became very involved in my drum shop and studio. I started to build a pretty good collection of students, spent many hours teaching and writing drum study books. I was oblivious to the world around me and possibly didn't pay much attention to my marriage. I probably should have and would have known more about that phase of my life.

As I look back, no one in my family told me much about sex, women, and all that went with this part of maturing. Well, my wife at that time was the business head of our family. I trusted her and she paid the bills and eventually we bought a house in Teaneck, New Jersey, and I was doing "the commuting thing," by car and later by bus. I was very involved in playing the club date scene and weddings and other special events that go with that phase of the music business.

The next thing I knew, we had all the credit cards one eventually gets. I found myself working hard and always paying off credit cards. I still didn't understand this but I figured it was part of being married and building a family. Pay, pay, pay.

As the years went by, I started to pay better attention to credit cards and debts. I really didn't like it. In the back of my mind, I wanted to get rid of this part of being married. Everyone was doing it and so I kept letting it slide. When I got divorced, I took the bull by the horns. I called the credit card people and told them I didn't want to have these cards any longer. I then set out to pay the dollars I owed, and finally got this monkey off my back.

It was so refreshing to have no credit cards, less and less debt, and finally I didn't owe anybody a thing. If I wanted something, I paid for it by check or with cash but I didn't run up any debts. NONE THEN and NONE NOW. Now I do understand that credit cards can be valuable when you travel or have a car, own a house, etc. Credit cards that are free of unpaid balances show that your credit is good. I saw that there were times when flashing a credit card was helpful. However I didn't like it for me, and so it was NO MORE FOR SAM.

It's nice not to owe dollars and have people chase you to collect the money by letters, telephone calls, and everything that goes with having credit cards. I just didn't want to owe anybody. No one duns me . . . meaning no one is hounding me for the dollars I owe them. It's a beautiful feeling. Some people flash a gang of credit cards because it is fashionable and then think people are impressed. I wasn't impressed with owing others my bucks.

SAM IS FREE OF THE CREDIT CARD CRAZE. If it's okay for you, then that's your thing, but as you get older and take a good look at the credit card world you'll see that I'm right. Anyway, it's right for SAM ULANO.

MODERATION, MODERATION, I SAY. TAKE IT EASY, STAY WITHIN YOUR MEANS AND BOUNDARIES. You'll be a happy person and just maybe you'll be able to do what you wish with your life. Amen.

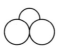

I Never Read Other Books About Philosophies of Life

M aybe the reason I am ABLE TO WRITE THIS COLLECTION OF MY THOUGHTS ABOUT MY LIFE is that I didn't get influenced by what the great philosophers wrote. Up to now I still haven't familiarized myself with what these people wrote. Maybe I should have.

I have heard from others what the great minds have said. They probably have said many important things that can help us understand our lives and where we are going. I am certain that their writings have a big effect on many of us. By the way, I don't call myself a "philosopher." I am just the average "Joe Public," saying what I feel I'VE LEARNED THROUGH THE YEARS AND WHERE I AM AT THIS STAGE OF MY LIFE.

I am not telling people how to live or what they should do with themselves. I am telling others how I have lived my life, how I take care of my body and my mind, what I would like to do with my life, and how I am following my dreams and desires. Maybe it is a diary of my life, past and present.

To me, some of the things I have lived by and still live by make sense. I see that this can bring results. I use a great deal of these concepts in my drum education with my students and I can see that it has helped.

My students don't do it exactly as I do it but they can feed off what I have been teaching and saying to them. As I look back, none of my drum educators played a big part in my life. None of them cared if I was getting fat or getting myself into good physical shape. None wondered how I practiced, how I studied, and what I wanted to do with my career in percussion.

When I wrote a book about drumming and showed it to my educators, none of them cared or were interested in what the book was about. Most of my instructors skimmed over what I showed them. I got no comments about whether the material had merit and possibly was something that might be valuable in drum study. This sort of took some "steam" out of me. But I was strong enough to believe in my work and knew I was doing something that could possibly be used by other drum students and teachers.

Since I liked what I was doing, I didn't care what my educators said about my work's potential. Maybe they were jealous of my talent to write and create new ideas that could be important in later years.

So as I write this, I realize that despite the fact that I didn't read the great philosophy books that were on the shelves in the library, I find that I have a pure mind, and my own thoughts are what are developing in these pages. This makes me feel good. Maybe later on in my life, I'll read other philosophies.

Do You Take Life Too Seriously?

Are you someone who takes life so seriously that it becomes unbearable, and you have a problem dealing with the daily routine of your life? I never understood what was so difficult in this life of ours that makes trying to get through each day of our lives a problem. Do you live every day with the feeling life is not worth living? What happens in your life that there isn't any fun in getting up in the morning and trying to make things work?

As I grew up day to day, year to year, and lived my life to the fullest, I found there wasn't anything that was too difficult to get through each day. I never found anything so terrible that I couldn't handle it. I would wake up each day and say, "THANK YOU, GOD, I hope you will allow me to work through my day and try to complete what I am working on."

I never took life so seriously that I couldn't work one day to the next. In fact, I had so much fun navigating through the hours of every day. The challenge of each hour and day was what was interesting to me. I know others have a problem with this concept of life. It's so great to be able to get up and say, "I am alive and I have something to look forward to."

Each day brings momentum to whatever I am thinking about and anticipating. TRY, TRY, TRY, I say to myself. "Sam, do this, do that, get things in order in your life." This is what I see life to be about . . . getting and keeping my life organized.

There are some days that I don't need to work on anything. Still, I believe in having everything in place so I don't have to rush through the day if everything gets jammed up to the point where I am choking myself with the mountain of work that has to be done.

There is nothing that makes life so serious that we must fight each day, day after day. Of course, I know there are many of us who find each day very difficult and somehow can't get things done. When I have days like that, I sit back, listen to some good music, and take life one day at a time. Each day, little by little, the serious things can be worked out.

No way are things so complicated that we have to see life as not worth living. Give yourself a fighting chance. I say to myself, "SAM ULANO, NOW AT EIGHTY-TWO YEARS OF AGE, JUST LOOK AT LIFE AS FUN AND WORTH PUTTING FULL EFFORT INTO."

Live life to have fun. That's my motto.

If You Succeed, All of the Credit Goes to You

always say when things don't come out right, we have ourselves to blame. However, on the other hand, if you succeed, you are the one to get the credit. I think that's only fair. We must take responsibility for our success or failure.

Don't be too bashful to take the rewards for your successes.

I like the feeling I get when I have positive results, and people give me credit for what I have done. That's how it should be. My years of working hard at my craft entitle me to the rewards that come with success. Don't be overly modest and say to people that what you've done is not so great.

Sometimes I have been blamed for being too pushy, and I may have been called greedy, because I am not ashamed to take the acclaim for what I do and am doing. I say, why shouldn't one get recognized for what they have done? So I say, if I succeed, I should get the credit. If there are others involved who have helped me succeed, I want to give them some of the credit for their involvement.

In writing my first book of my philosophy at age eighty, Ed Petoniak did the editing. He deserves the credit for helping me make this book read well. He made corrections as he saw them and did what an editor does. I am sure you agree with this concept. Give credit where credit is due.

My publisher also gets credit for making the book look very smart and professional. I may have planted the seeds of ideas about how the book should be set up but those who do the printing, editing, and cover design must enjoy the fruits of their efforts.

When I see a record or CD produced with no photo of the band and no mention of the people who recorded the CD, I think this is not nice. Many times my students will bring me a CD with some cover drawing or a picture of trees, or the sky or something that has nothing to do with the CD. I go "bananas," because I don't know what the members of the band look like and sometimes I don't even know what instruments these people play.

Give credit to all who deserve it. Let the world know who you are. Let them know what part you played in developing the book, article, CD, or film. It's healthy and good for our egos. I like to be noticed. I like it when I can present my work, and everyone knows I am either the creator or someone who helped create the project.

Don't Borrow Money . . . You'll Be Sorry

I am glad I learned that borrowing money was dangerous. Not a smart thing to do. Yes, I know there are times that you need money. These are events that we must consider. For me, I avoid borrowing money from friends or banks or a credit card, whatever the borrowing form might be. I hate to owe dollars and I hate to have to be on a schedule to pay back the loan.

When I want to do something and don't have enough money to finance whatever I need it for, I try to save it up until I have enough dollars to go ahead with the purchase. Does this make sense to you? Putting myself in debt can be a problem. So I give you my reasons for not jumping the gun to finance the project. Complete the project later rather than hurrying into owing someone and tying yourself up.

When I have the money in place and can move ahead, I then set my project in motion and make plans to do what I want to do. In the long run, I always find I am happier because I eventually get my work done with no strings attached. This is my way of doing things without tying my hands and being beholden to others.

Sometimes a little patience and waiting until I can afford what I wish keeps my mind relaxed and happy. I owe no one, and when I do my "thing," I pay for it. It's more fun doing these things, for me.

Others see that borrowing money will allow them time to produce what they see as important. Recently a student of mine spent four or five thousand dollars fixing up his drum studio, never getting permission from his landlord. After having all of this work done and paying for it, his landlord sold the building and the new owners wanted him to leave. They also sued him for doing things to the property without permission. Guess what? He lost the case; the judge ruled in favor of the new owners and my student was stuck with the bill to restore the property. He had borrowed quite a bit of money to do this renovation and was paying back the original loan and now he had to find the dollars to restore the property.

So borrowing bucks can be a problem and can tie you up for quite a while. NOT A GOOD POLICY. NOT GOOD FOR YOU. Stay away from borrowing dollars. Do things when you have the money.

If You Are in Charge, Be in Charge

I always say, if you are the person who directs a special project, you should take full command of whatever has to be done. Someone has to run the operation, and since it is you, then you must be in full charge. NO IFS, ANDS, OR BUTS. You cannot shirk your duties in this type of situation.

When I was the bandleader at the RED BLAZER, I hired the men in the band, gave everyone in the band directions about when we start to play, and what kind of event might take place at the club. I tried to arrange for some supper for the band members. I dealt with management and collected the band's pay and paid each member.

I take full charge. If there are problems, I try to solve them. When I book a band, I tell them how we will dress and call the names of the songs we will play throughout the evening. I tell the band when we will break and when we will be back on the bandstand. There is no one else in the band who takes charge. I also handle requests from the audience and have the band play these requests.

If there is no one in charge, then it would be like an ARMY without a GENERAL. In business, someone runs the office, someone makes sure things run smoothly. Big business has a chain of command: it could start with the president of the company, the vice president, then the office manager, and go all the way down to the workers. COMPANY COMMAND HAS TO HAVE THIS KIND OF SYSTEMATIC ORGANIZATION. It's the only way the company can function.

I'm a big believer that things must run this way. Each of us has to do our thing, TAKE DIRECTION and FOLLOW ORDERS. It makes sense to me.

Throughout my early years and eventually in my professional life, the conductor of an orchestra was in charge all of the time. As an instructor, I am in charge at my studio. I teach my students that they eventually will have to take direction from me. Someone has to be in charge. In baseball, football, basketball, and most sports, there is someone who directs the team. The "top dog" runs things. That's how it is and that is how it must be. Otherwise we would have disaster.

If you are married, you and your wife are IN CHARGE OF THE HOUSE, AND THE FINANCES. THE CHILDREN HAVE TO BE TAUGHT TO FOLLOW ORDERS AND THEN THE HOUSEHOLD CAN FUNCTION. The parents are the head of the home. This is how it should be.

As the years move on we should learn something about our lives and how to run them. Simple as that. I see that someone must be always in charge. No other way will provide the answer to how things can and should be done. That's how I see it.

How Do You Feel About Retiring?

This is an interesting thought. Eventually we all will have to give retirement our utmost attention. I hear all kinds of views about what people are going to do when and if they reach this phase of their lives. You can't escape it. It is inevitable. It presents a challenge to all of us: We must decide how we are going to handle finishing our life's work, whatever it is. This is something that there has been a great deal written about.

Each of us have our own thoughts about what we will do and how we will do it when retirement time comes. Some of us work in a field where the company says we must retire, possibly at the age of fifty-five or sixty-five, but this is the corporate idea of when it's time to retire. Some of us get a special amount of money to leave a job; others get a watch or some token from the company, or they might have a party for us when we are ready to leave. There are many ways it happens.

You have to ask yourself, ARE YOU READY TO RETIRE? What are your feelings about leaving a job that you loved and enjoyed for many years? Sometimes we hate the job and can't wait to get out of there, or we might have made a gang of wonderful friends but are forced to leave because it is a company rule.

How are you preparing for your retirement years? Have you saved enough dollars? Will you look for another job if you are still young and have the strength and desire to keep working? Many of us might open a little business; many may finally travel around the world — a trip that we would have loved to do earlier but were in a very special job and couldn't leave. Now that we are moving on, we must give some thought to what we wish to do and how we will do it.

If you are in good health and like golf, you might join a golf club and find happiness in improving your game. I don't know if this works for you, since we all have different ideas on how we will handle this new approach to life.

I have asked many friends what they plan to do when they retire. I want to know their concept of the next phase of life. Will they take a year off and then decide what to do with all of this free time? Some get a good pension and have enough dollars to do what they want to do. If they have kids, how will this fit into their new setup? A great deal of thinking about all of this should be done while we are young and APPROACHING THE RETIREMENT STAGE OF OUR LIVES.

DO YOU WANT TO RETIRE? HOW DO YOU FEEL YOU'D LIKE TO GO ON WITH YOUR LIFE? DO YOU HAVE AN IDEA WHAT YOU WANT FROM YOUR LIFE WHEN THIS TIME COMES? HAVE YOU MADE PLANS? THINK, THINK, THINK ABOUT IT and maybe you'll know what you want.

My Concepts About Retiring

At eighty-two, I have given this business of retiring much thought. I have a big problem with this, because, at my age I still love my music and work as much, if not more, than ever. I can't give up the one thing that has given, and still gives me, so much joy and pleasure.

How do you just stop doing what has rewarded you every day of your life? May I say that right now, I can't see ending this beautiful relationship with my daily existence. I don't want to give it up.

Why should I? How would I replace it? I have no idea what will make my days so enjoyable other than what I've done all my life. I find that the more I play my drums and stay involved with all aspects of music, the happier I am.

And to tell you the truth, I still have so much to learn. I can get better and improve my drum playing. I can play a couple of nights a week with my band. I feel there are things to write about that have not been covered and I would like to be the person that writes about them and develops material that has not been documented for drummers.

There is so much to investigate and develop. I just can't see giving up and not staying in my field.

I might write another hundred books, produce new CDs, videos and much more. I think I can practice and develop new techniques. I have a mind that is fresh and fertile — capable of discovering so much more. I know I can do it.

If retiring is your cup of tea, so be it. It's not for me and I can't see myself thinking of it. I am full of life and even at eighty-two, going on eighty-three, I have a lot to live for and more to give of my talents.

When I hear people talk about being at the end of their working days and wanting to take it easy, I say to myself, "Sam, you have so much more to do, so don't listen to these people and don't even think the way they do."

I LOVE WHAT I DO and will go on loving what I am doing.

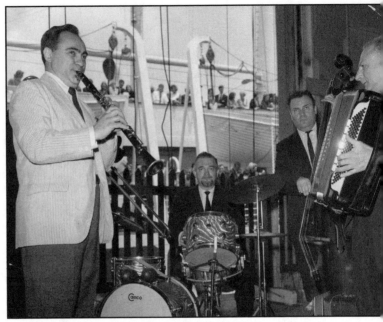

Sam backing Sol Yaged, 1960 on a jazz cruise ship
NOTE: Sol taught Steve Allen to impersonate Benny
Goodman for the movie, *The Benny Goodman Story*.

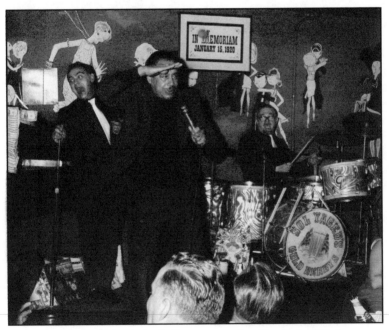

Sam and Sol with Cab Calloway at the Gaslight Club,
NYC, 1966

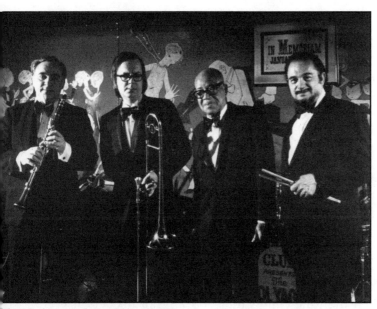

The Sol Yaged Quartet, 1973
Photograph courtesy of Raymond Ross, NYC

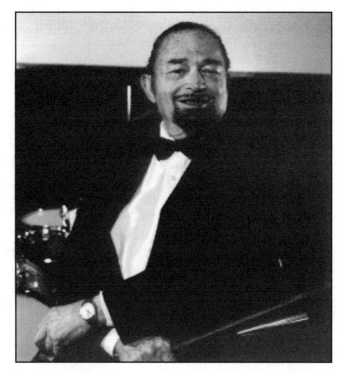

Sam Ulano, December 2002

You Know You're Old When You Retire

In my mind, when people think about retiring, I say it's a sign that you are getting old and life is passing you by. Of course, this is only my opinion and doesn't mean it's true. I just feel that it's a sign that we have lost the purpose and drive for living unless you are someone who has developed an idea as to what you want to do with yourself.

At a young age, you should develop a plan as to what you want to do with your current days and future years. Of course, as you get older, you should think hard about what you will do with your life when the time comes that you are not needed at your job.

I guess I shouldn't be the one discussing this business of ending my regular job and moving on to the next phase of my life, because I am an unusual case. At the young age of thirteen, I found what I love to do. People like myself can't speak for others; however, I have formulated a definite plan as to how I want my older years to play out.

Since I love what I do and enjoy my life so much, I realize how lucky I am. I don't know if it's luck, because I've spent a lifetime developing my talents in my field. I am one of the few people I know who has stuck with their dream. This makes my daily life happy and gives me something to look forward to each day. I know I will be doing my thing. I can practice and study and know what I am after so this is what it is about, for me.

Yet, I still think when we retire we are getting old. I hope you who read this will not be satisfied to sit on your butt, watching television, overeating, and just letting your life roll by. If and when you retire, see if you can make a better effort to improve your life and see if you can set up a definite plan for your older years. You'll be happier if you do make this plan and carry it out.

Just don't feel you are old because you have retired. You are not old, you're just going into the next stage of your life. Since you have better control of your older years, it's a chance to do some of the things you had planned for yourself.

We shouldn't let our older years slip away without having a desire to stay in good health and improve our bodies. This is important so that we don't get discouraged with our lives. You can do it. In fact, I have been doing it so I will continue to love what I do. YES, I WILL CONTINUE TO LOVE WHAT I DO.

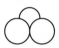

Only You Can Tell How You Feel
While You're Getting Older

Only you can feel the pain of a blister. Only you can say how you feel today. You're the only one who can tell the doctor where it hurts. Only you can tell the dentist which tooth is giving you the most problems. Think about this: You are the only person who knows how you feel as you are getting older.

Someone knows you are having a birthday and asks you how it feels to be fifty (or whatever). You are the person who knows how you feel from one birthday to the next. You then can answer, "I don't feel any different."

I once wrote a friend who asked me how I feel now that I am approaching eighty-three. I said, "I feel wonderful and I am so glad that I took care of myself all these years, since my fortieth birthday, back in 1960." George Burns, the great comedian, when he reached one hundred years of age, said that had he known he was going to live this long he would have taken better care of himself. Great line.

We are the ones who should be able to take care of ourselves. If we are not in the best shape now, we should try to imagine what it will be like as we get on in years. For myself, I want to feel the best I can as the years roll on, so I have come up with this concept that I have been writing about in my PHILOSOPHY OF LIFE. I'm very serious about this: I would be very unhappy had I not had the wisdom, the desire, and the intelligence to make every effort to understand my body and work at staying in excellent physical shape.

As we get older, various aches and pains start to show up: ARTHRITIS, CANCER, ALL THE VARIOUS DISEASES THAT ARE KNOWN TO ATTACK THE BODY. By working on our health and using our minds, we can develop a concept as to just how we wish to keep our body in shape and eventually find that the hard work has paid off, and we are ready to move into this major phase of our lives.

Getting old can be fun. Getting old can also be a drag. If we don't take care for ourselves, we become susceptible to all kinds of serious aches and pains. What do we want to happen to us as these years come if we are not on top of our game? This has to be planned out and the plan followed.

Of course, if we are not in the best of shape, we might find getting on in years not the most exciting part of living. In a discussion with some friends of mine, we found that each person had a different idea of how to treat his or her retirement years.

There Are Many Advantages To Being a Senior

Once I had passed sixty years of age, I started to realize that I was really approaching my senior years, and it made me wonder how I would feel about getting on in years. It's interesting that most people get a bit frightened of growing older, and they start to worry about how they will handle this part of their lives. Some, of course, never make it past sixty.

In my mind, I understand why I was so happy at this time of my life. I was approaching my social security benefits, and I was also very involved with my music, teaching, and writing about drumming. I still was very active in performing with my band and in other musical situations. All of this made me feel great. Just think what you can do in your later years. If you took care in your earlier years, you just might be ready to enter your senior years in good shape.

If you don't have a serious illness and still have good hearing and eyesight, if your mental attitude is positive and happy, you will be able to do a lot of the things you love to do. This is a wonderful way to reach your senior years.

If your reflexes are sharp and you have good control of your legs, all of this helps you to function as you would like to function. One important thing to remember is that you are not a youngster any longer and things you could do at twenty or thirty are not part of you now. So keep in mind that you have to adjust your concept of what you are capable of doing after the age of sixty. Once you realize this, you will then have learned one of the great lessons of your life.

Being a senior means that you can ride buses at half-price. The price of a movie ticket is also better, and people treat you with a different respect. If you are in a special field, many of your friends make you into a "guru." You might give younger people information they could only get from living and younger people will find you are very valuable in their lives.

I find now that I am eighty-two, people in my industry feel I have some valuable ideas to pass on to them. My students come and take my instruction very seriously. They treat me with profession-al attitudes. They know they can learn from me and I can back up what I teach them. They respect that I have the practical experi-ence to help the student grow into a potential percussionist.

As a senior who has been involved for years with my drum abil-ity, I have my students study hard. They become better drum-mers and can develop as serious players.

This part of your senior life is what makes being older more fun. It's one of the rewards of being a senior.

I Have Lived in a Senior Citizen Center for the Past Sixteen Years

I have been fortunate to live in a Senior Center here in New York City. These past years have been a great lesson for me. I have learned to appreciate my older years and respect the fact that growing older becomes a great education.

Here are some of the things I have learned living in the Senior Center: Take care of your body first. I do my exercises and don't try to do things that are now more difficult to do. I have learned that I must get my sleep and can't dissipate myself. I take good care of my clothing and laundry. I know I must eat with a definite system. Living at the Center, I see that I have a chance to grow old gracefully. I can still study and keep on top of my talents with what I love to do.

I'm glad I never was drunk. I am so happy that many years ago I stopped smoking. I'm really happy that I don't overeat and feel that this has helped me keep my body weight under control. This is a very important lesson to learn as you become a senior.

I don't expect too much of myself at my age. However, since I have spent a lot of time preparing for my older years, I can enjoy these years now. Many seniors are enjoying their lives. They know that in their senior days they reap the rewards of earlier planning for this time of life.

I am enjoying my life now because it's fun when you're in good condition. This all depends on how you feel about some of the things I have been writing about. Give it some thought, and you too will come to the same conclusions I have.

Don't feel that as you get older there isn't much left for you, and all that is left is your life ending. I can speak from experience that my life is fun, first because I am still doing what I love and I still can use most of my talents. That makes me happy and it makes a lot of sense. Living in a Senior Center, I meet a lot of people in my age bracket. These seniors have a lot to say about their past and how they are coping now that they too are "up there" in age. I'm enjoying the Senior Center. It's just great.

Don't Be Afraid of Growing Older

Some people I have met tell me that they are afraid of growing older. I ask them, "What is there to be afraid of, and why worry about it?" It's not that bad. In fact, it should be fun. Of course, if you don't have your mind occupied, if you don't have anything to live for, if you are still living in the past, this can make one a bit frightened about approaching their senior years. I can sympathize with how these people feel.

Sometimes, as we get older, we get lonely. We start to feel sorry for ourselves. Some seniors are not physically well. They have medical problems and maybe their bodies are not in the best of shape. This can be difficult to live with. It would be a good idea to get involved with someone who can give you some ideas as to how to train. Even though you are growing older, there still are some simple exercises you can do. This certainly can help you get your body back in shape.

There is nothing you can do about getting older. It is all a definite part of life. As they say, "it goes with the territory." You can't stop the days and years from moving on.

Find a good nutritionist to teach you how to eat properly, and stick with the program. Have your doctor help you take better care of your body and your mental attitude. That can be very valuable to you. Taking care of yourself is one of the answers to feeling well and making your older years fun to live. This can encourage you to grow older feeling good.

At eighty-two, I see only the bright side of being "up there" in my life. I must "go with the flow." What you want out of your older years will depend on your approach to your senior years. I feel I've "got it made," because I worked at staying in excellent condition.

If you are young and reading my Philosophy of Life, heed my advice and start taking good care of yourself. You will stand a better chance of reaching your senior days — and enjoying them — if you get on top of being in good shape. It will pay off in the long run.

So I say once again, "Don't be afraid of getting older. DON'T WORRY, BECAUSE IT WON'T HELP A BIT."

Have You Given Up on Your Desires?

Have you found as you are getting older you have given up on all of your desires? Have you lost your love for things you used to love to do?

Or is the fire still burning in your heart for what you love to do? Sometimes we get older and we lose our desires. That's too bad, my friends, because doing what we really love is one of the greatest parts of living our lives. I think we should keep the flames burning in our hearts and minds. Then, even if we lose some of that drive for what we love, I think we should try to fan the flames and see if we can rekindle the excitement.

For myself, I'm looking forward to what I will be doing at eighty-three. Maybe I'll see something special that I really want to accomplish and can look forward to working on. Then I'll say to myself, yeah, that's it. For now, I'll put the final touches on whatever it is I am currently working on.

Just recently, I found a manuscript that I wrote about four or five years ago. I was cleaning out some of my shelves of ideas. Boom! This piece of work struck my eyes and mind and I said, "This is good. Why didn't I complete it?"

This was like a new look at the material and more ideas came to me. I made up a title, cleaned up the pages of study material, wrote an introduction and an explanation of what the book was about, and bingo! the book has been doing well. Teachers and students dig it the most.

I called this book *THE INSANITY DRUM READER* and the photo on the cover sure fits the title.

I never throw away ideas that I may have worked on many years before, because this has happened to me so often. The drive to complete what I started some time in the past gets going once again. I'm certain many of you out there have experienced this phenomenon. KEEP YOUR MIND, BRAIN, HEART DESIRES BURNING. MAYBE THE SECOND TIME AROUND, AS THE SONG SAYS, "LOVE (OR LIFE) IS LOVELIER . . ."

It's funny, now at age eighty-two, I find so many things that I started earlier come back to me once again. I can't give you reasons why, but I'm so amazed at the way this has been happening to me in my life. Don't sell yourself short. If your mind and computer brain seem to hit a stone wall, you never know, maybe the next look at what you were working on will make more sense to you. Like a lot of us, I try not to throw away working ideas. Not just yet.

Have You Become a "Couch Potato?"

Someone who sits on his or her butt and watches TV many hours of the day, doing nothing with their lives, has been called a COUCH POTATO. To me this is terrible. In my life I sort of classify this as a form of sickness: allowing your life to rot away and having nothing to do to fill all these wonderful hours. How can you allow this to happen to your body and mind?

I say, WAKE UP, get started on something. There are lots of young people who find themselves wasting away, day by day, week by week, year by year. Just awful. Of course, I can understand why this happens to many of us when we shut our brains down. Unless you give yourself a wake-up shock, the brain gets dull.

If you fit into the category of being a COUCH POTATO, start thinking about what's happening to you.

In my philosophy of life, I have no place for this kind of existence. My television time is limited. Maybe I'll watch about an hour a week, maybe two hours. Some weeks I never turn my television set on at all. I have so much to do with my life. To allow even a precious hour to dissipate, to melt away, with nothing accomplished? Man, I'd kick my butt or get someone to kick my ASS.

I call this a waste of good time. A dead brain. I think people who are going through this phase of their lives are very sick people.

Someone said we must get up, go out, and smell the roses. Take a walk and think about this life you are leading: DOING NOTHING IS LOSING A GRIP ON YOUR TALENTS. Yes, I know you worked hard all of your life and are entitled to relax and just let everyone else do all the hard work.

Think of this: The world and all its people don't give a rap about what you do with yourself. They don't care if you are not participating in something. Only you know what is going on with your life. Many times we overeat, do little or no body training, just rot away. This is so bad for you.

This is why I have been writing my concept of what I am doing with my life. I try to cover all the bases. Study, improve my talents, think about what is next in store for me, how I can play my drums better. I answer my mail, make telephone calls, practice and practice more. I review every day and stick to my body conditioning routine. There are hundreds of things I think about and then think again.

DON'T BE A COUCH POTATO, MY FRIENDS. YOU WILL BE WASTING YOUR LIFE. NOT TOO GOOD FROM WHERE I SIT. YOU MUST MAKE THE DECISION.

Where Will You Spend Your Retirement Years?

Where will you want to go when and if you retire? Some of us want to go to Florida, some to Arizona, some to California. There are so many places. However, the question is, when you retire, will you find the place where you will want to spend your senior years? For myself, I will not go to any of the above parts of the U.S. I need to be in a place where I can be active and keep my mind occupied.

If and when I do decide to retire, I can't see myself being in any other place than New York. In New York I don't need a car. In New York I will have places to play music and stay on top of my talents. I do a lot of writing, so I need a printer or printing facility nearby and I need the kind of people that can accommodate me. Since I won't give up my teaching practice, I will have to have a studio and a place where students can get to me right away.

So what I'm saying to you is I'll be retired and yet I won't be retired. I always tell everyone that I have been retired even in my younger days. I hate the thought of not being active. My concept of being retired is that I want to keep doing what I love. I just want to stay active as a senior person. My whole life has been active and if I stop doing what I love, I'll be one of the unhappiest human beings in this world.

Crazy, isn't it? Everyone I know can't wait to retire and get away from whatever they did during their career. They want to really retire; to travel, visit relatives, different things. Not I. I have too much fun doing my thing. So all in all, I just haven't got the desire to stop what has made me happy. I'm a bit selfish. I want to keep going.

I hate the thought of saying I'm retired. I have always said that I never intend to retire. Thus I've never considered a retirement location. My favorite line that I say to everyone when the subject of retiring comes up is, "I'm a person that has been retired all my life." I have been lucky because, as I wrote in Book One, my vocation has also been my avocation.

As I Get Older, I Must Have Fun with My Life

Earlier I told you what my Mom always said: she would remind all of her children that every day they should have a good time with their lives. She used to say, "You have to enjoy every day and have lots of fun. If you don't enjoy every day, then there is something wrong with your life. You must be doing something wrong and you'd better try to correct it."

My Mother was a very wise person, and I inherited this idea from her, because now I realize she knew what she was talking about. There is enough misery in this world. Who needs more of it? We must learn to laugh. We must take each day as it comes and work at being happy and loving our daily existence.

My Mom was so right. In fact, most of the time she was right. There are twenty-four hours in each day, seven days in a week, and fifty-two weeks in a year, and it's my feeling that each one of those days I must make myself happy. If I can be happy with people, that's even better. I read the newspapers every day and there are so many disasters that happen and it's a sad day that we have to read these papers that give us horrible news. So what can we do about it?

For myself, I work at having a wonderful day every day. I look up to God and say, "Thanks for a good night's sleep," and also thank Him for helping me to feel great. I then tell the Lord that I am going to have a beautiful day and that with His help I'll get through each day. These are my first thoughts every day. After I have done my morning exercise, lifted my weights, taken my medication, visited the bathroom, bathed, and dressed, I head to my studio. After a good breakfast, if the Post Office is open, I get my mail and buy stick-on postage stamps. I accumulate stamps because many times I have to do a mailing.

I again thank God if the weather is wonderful and think how great it is to be alive, having Him watch over me. You may call it praying or whatever. (Maybe it's talking to myself.) But I like my own company, and all of this fits so marvelously together. When I reach my studio, I do about two hours of drum reading practice. I do this seven days a week, unless I start a few lessons in the morning. After the lessons, I then do my own practice. I take an hour to work on my writing.

All of this put together helps me enjoy each day. My days must be full and I must enjoy life and have fun. There's no other way for me. I don't know about you out there, but life has to be sensational for me. I am the only one that can make it so. NO ONE ELSE WILL DO THIS FOR YOU. Take it from me, life should be happy and fun for you. You are in control.

THINK ABOUT IT AND MAKE IT WORK.

Don't Live Only for Your Kids

Kids are great. They are probably the greatest miracle of all time. If you don't believe in miracles, then you have a problem. I have always believed in this part of life. We are miracles . . . a child is born, grass grows, birds and bees, all that fantastic stuff. Even the lowly cockroach is one of the wonders of this world. They were here long before all of us and are still going, and from what I read, they will be here long after we are gone.

Having children is one of the most fantastic things in the world. They are born and grow up to be like us; they eventually leave us and start their own wonderful world. I am a big believer that we can do the best for our kids keeping in mind that we come first. I've written this before, but I must tell you how I feel about kids. We are first. Kids come next. If you don't see this, you will sacrifice yourself and life can become miserable.

We can enjoy the children when they are born and grow into such beauty. Yes, they are wonderful to have, but eventually they go to school, high school, then college. When they get married, they may rely on the love of Mom and Pop, but they must learn to fend for themselves, make their own bucks, support their own lives, just as we did. It starts all over again and the big "kicker" here is that if they start to depend on you, eat into your hard-earned dollars, man, you're at their mercy. If you allow them, they will eat you out of house and home, make a dent in your dollars, and negatively affect your existence.

I believe in letting our young ones learn how to support themselves. Let them support their own kids, wife, girlfriends. A friend for many years said to me, YOU COME FIRST AND THAT IS HOW IT SHOULD BE. If you don't come first, you will be sorry. Take it from me, YOU FIRST.

Yes, "YOU COME FIRST" IS A VERY SELFISH STATEMENT, I know; but for you to grow older and be able to handle your senior years, you have to take a stand in your life. YOU FIRST means you can take care of you. What you wish to contribute to your kids is up to you yourself.

Some friends of mine have spoiled their kids rotten. They gave their kids everything. I WANT MY KIDS TO HAVE EVERYTHING THAT I DIDN'T HAVE AS A YOUNGSTER. It's so nice to say this, but it will eventually destroy you. Kids don't make a marriage. KIDS DON'T MAKE EVERYTHING GREAT.

When I left my home in Teaneck, New Jersey, I went on with my life. If I saw my young ones, it was okay. There would be times the kids and I never saw each other. I lived, did my thing, and enjoyed my life. I never felt I had to be with my children every day, twenty-four hours a day. Now that my son is forty-seven and my daughter is about forty-two, I talk to them on the telephone. They're busy. I'm busy. But we make contact and life goes on.

You Have To Be a Bit Selfish

I think that if we are to do the things we love and wish to accomplish some degree of success in what we want in our lives, we must be selfish. Or, let me say, we must "do our thing" first. The way I see it is that if we take care of ourselves first we can take care of other things in our life.

At eighty-two, I know more than ever that I was right. With a bit of a greedy, selfish, ME FIRST attitude, I now see that I got a great deal done and that is what made me happy and very satisfied. I really think all people who have succeeded in their lives had this same feeling. I needed hours to do everything I was reaching for and so my hours and concentration were directed inwardly. I can say, I was very selfish. I put all of my free hours into my development. I look back now and see I was smart to think this way.

How far did I carry this selfish life? To the fullest. And here I am, still thinking the same way. I still have too much to do, so I have to stay on this track. ME FIRST, EVERYTHING ELSE IS SECONDARY. I wrote *I Love What I Do!* with hard work. Every day for nine days and then it was completed. Once I had finished the first draft and gave it to my editor, I had lots of free time. I also had a nice book that I could show to people and, of course, the events that followed led to its publication. Now it is in print and available to the reading public.

This showed me that some selfishness can be very rewarding. I have said and have written that you can't get anything done unless you work at it. I feel it's okay, as long as I put my efforts into the things I love and it doesn't hurt others. I just use my hours for myself. I tell all of my students that they must put time in on their training and practice and work very hard TO GET THE RESULTS THAT WE ARE AFTER. I tell them all, nothing happens unless we make it happen.

My son, Mark Ulano, who is involved with the film industry and does the sound for many pictures, said to me a number of times that I was selfish, ONLY THINKING OF MYSELF. Maybe so, but now that he is forty-seven years old and is working hard in his field, he has told me, he understands very well now that it was the only way I could reach my goals. This is because he too had to be selfish to accomplish what he has done in his business.

DON'T BE SORRY IF YOU ARE SELFISH. THIS IS HOW WE GET THINGS DONE.

Study Yourself As You Get Older

I always say we live with ourselves. Even if you are married or
have a live-in partner, if you have kids or live with your family from birth, we must study ourselves, decide what makes us
tick, and learn what we can about ourselves.

I know that when I was younger I didn't think this way. I didn't
know much about me. I started to love drumming at the age of
thirteen, but never knew why. I didn't enjoy school but didn't
have the faintest idea why I didn't like to study. I remember I
loved to play stickball with my friends and always loved to listen
to all kinds of music.

When I was aware of the big band era, I started to like listening
to BASIE, ELLINGTON, BENNY, and the other bands that were
broadcasting on the various radio stations. I even started to collect some 78 RPM recordings. I recall my eldest brother, Al, talking about Louis Armstrong and Duke Ellington's band. Al was
involved with music in his early days. He played violin and some
trumpet but he never really stuck with it.

In our family, Al was sort of a "MAVEN" (an authority) about
music, and everyone in the family respected his opinions about
the music world. As I got older and started to teach and perform
and write some of my first drum instruction books, I became a bit
of an authority about music too. I was fascinated by the study of
music and the practicing of my instrument.

I started to find out more about myself as I got up there in years.
I changed a lot of my habits. I discovered something about myself
when it came to sex. I really loved that part of my growing years.
As I knew more about how I felt about loving someone, I realized
that I had to be more of a giver. I wasn't much of a taker, but I'm
certain as I matured, I knew that love was a beautiful part of living my life.

Now that I'm advancing to eighty-three years of age, I know a great deal about my likes and dislikes. I know more about my inner feelings. It's wonderful to understand who I am and what makes SAM ULANO who he is. I think we all should study ourselves and this could make us so happy. It's great when this happens. I know it has happened to me. I love it.

Set Up a Purpose for Yourself

I always say we can't go anywhere without knowing where we are going. If you never have been where you are going and don't know how to get there, you either get a map that shows you the way or get directions from someone who has been there. Of course, that is easier said than done, but what I am really saying is we must have a reason and purpose for where we are heading. This makes sense to me, and I think it should make sense to you. Having a purpose for what you wish to do and following that purpose might just give you the ideas you need to accomplish what you'd like.

What are you after? What do you plan to do with what you are working on? Is what you are setting up in your mind really something that you love to do? Will it be something that you will love to do all of your life? When I set my sights on teaching the drums, I knew from the start it was something I loved. When I was young, I never thought that I would be doing this all my living days, but I had an idea and a feeling that I was going to fall in love with music.

The driving force to do what I love was burning inside of me and the flames became stronger as the years went on. Once I had realized my purpose to play my drums, I developed the love that has been with me all these years.

I set up a plan that was what I wanted to do and where I wanted to go with the talent I have to play with bands, teach others, and carry this on throughout my life. Do you want to know something? IT PROVED TO BE TRUE. Those of you who are reading my thoughts should think about your life and study yourself. You should ask yourself, "What am I after?"

HOW WILL YOU KEEP THE FIRES BURNING IN YOUR MIND, HEART, AND BRAIN? What will stir you up? How will you follow your path to success? Will you always be ready to work every day on your talents? Can you see yourself "doing your thing" every day? How will you follow up each day with the thing you love?

The questions I present to you are not easy to answer. What I'm suggesting is that it takes a great deal of stick-to-it-ness. Every day should add to the day before and you should add a new piece to what your purpose is about.

It's like a flower. In order to grow it needs patience and care. It's the same with your goals.

Take Care of Your Eyes and Ears

Every day I wake up I tell myself that I must take care of my vision and hearing. This is a definite priority in my lifestyle. As I have been telling you throughout my writing, there are certain things that I have become very careful about, among them my eyesight and hearing. You and I would be lost without either our vision or our hearing. Many of us have become very neglectful about these two important parts of living.

Without my eyes, I would be lost. As a DIABETIC, I have become more aware of how much I must take care of my eyes. There are many diseases that affect our eyes. I have my eyes checked every month or so at the VETERANS HOSPITAL at 23rd Street and First Avenue, here in New York. They make sure that I have the correct glasses, that my diabetes is not affecting my eyesight. NO FOOLING AROUND.

Just recently, through extensive tests, they found that my hearing has lost a step or two and so they provided me with excellent hearing aids. I use them a few hours a day in theaters, in restaurants, and on other occasions that hearing aids can help me. This is so important in my work as well.

I tell all of my students, if they need glasses, get them. Don't give me the baloney that you don't think you look well with glasses. That's a hunk of nonsense. Get glasses if the doctors tell you that you should have them. As for hearing aids, I know quite a few people who should and must have hearing aids. Some tell me that they can't stand them and do not wish to get them. But it's very important.

I have them because a very lovely lady friend noticed that I had a slight hearing deficiency and suggested I have my hearing tested. The audiologist said I had about fifteen to twenty percent loss of hearing. This too was at the VA Hospital and, sure enough, I have hearing aids. They're very helpful under certain conditions.

I've learned this lesson well. I needed hearing aids. I got them. Simple as all that. Don't neglect your hearing and vision. You will regret it later on. Do it now. If you need glasses, make up your mind that you'll look great with glasses. If you need hearing aids, get them.

I am certain we all learn our lessons better as we get up there in age. Nothing wrong in having the proper treatment for your own good. Take a lesson from an old codger like me, guys and gals. Neglect can be detrimental to your well-being. No two ways about it. In the long run you'll think like I do. Catch it early and you'll be happy that you did. **DON'T WAIT.**

As You Get Older, You Will Experience the Same Things That All Seniors Do

Do you think you're any different than all the rest of us? Do you think you will not go through the life experiences most of us go through? What makes you think you are different than the next person, man or woman? No way. We all are born, all grow up one day at a time, go to school, fall in love, and experience all the same things. As a child, we have fun. As a teenager, we live through similar lifestyles as single people in their teens do. We grow into young adults, get married, have a few kids, and grow into our senior years. Before you know it, life is what it becomes as a senior.

I tell you this, if you haven't realized it, that your life is very much like the next person's. A lot depends on how we take care of ourselves, physically and educationally as we approach our senior years. If you learn your lessons well, you stand a great chance of enjoying these years, let's say between fifty-five and eighty-five. Of course, I don't know what is ahead for each of us, I can only talk about myself.

I think I was one of the lucky few who wakes up and smells the roses. I studied myself very seriously and here, at this ripe old age of eighty-two, going on eighty-three, I am in wonderful condition, mentally and physically. It's so great to be in wonderful shape. This, to me, is because I took care to make the effort that staying in shape requires. NO SHORTCUTS.

I can prove it to you. I AM VERY HEALTHY, NOT OVERWEIGHT ANY LONGER, I HAVE STAMINA, I HAVE A CLEAR MIND AND MY BRAIN, AS FAR AS I CAN SEE, IS IN BEAUTIFUL CONDITION.

I'm bragging, but I have a right to brag. My theory of life has worked. I don't have to look for the fountain of youth. IT'S IN MY MIND.

I Am So Lucky To Be Alive and Still Doing What I Love To Do

Some of my very close friends have said to me, "SAM, YOU'VE GOT IT MADE!" I say to them that I worked at it all these years, and I now am reaping the rewards for living my life as I have. Some of the important things I tell my buddies is that I have defeated STRESS. I have defeated problems with my stomach. I don't worry. I get no headaches. I get no back pains, no arthritis, no loss of memory. I got rid of skin cancer when they operated on me back in 1985 at the VA Hospital.

I don't call my lifestyle "luck." It was due to serious thinking on how to handle my life. I'm not a fanatic or hypochondriac, although some people seem to think I am. I listened to people who showed me the way. Sigmond Klein at his gym, for instance. He showed me the way to train my body. I listened to him and, lo and behold, his advice was very wonderful. All I had to do was follow it to the letter.

I listen to the advice of the medical people that I am involved with. They said to operate on my skin cancer and I allowed them to do it. Knock on wood, I no longer have skin cancer. I listened to and trusted these people. I also listened to my inner self. Practice and study. Train every day with a purpose and stay on top of my abilities. Simple as that.

I can't predict that my concepts of life will work for everyone. That is for sure. However, I see it working for me and so maybe, just maybe, it could work for others. You who are reading my philosophy of life might give it a try. Who knows, it may be the answer you are looking for.

Living and doing what I love to do to me seems to be a recipe for a healthy existence. If you love what you do in your daily life and it makes you happy and may help you reach some sort of success, why wouldn't you give it a try? My mother's advice was that life was too short and we should live it to the fullest. Take care of your body, take care of your mind, and educate yourself. To me, this makes so much sense.

Drugs, drinking, smoking, not getting sufficient sleep, not training yourself every day, letting your talents slip away all make up a very poor approach to what our lives are about. When I tell people I never was drunk they say, "Man, you sure have missed something." What, I don't know. As for experimenting with various drugs to see what it's like, to me that's nuts! I smoked and gave it up many years ago and have never missed it. What can I tell you? These vices seem to be too dangerous.

If it is for you, then fine, but not for Sam Ulano. You can have it. I'm not lucky. I think I'm smart. Very smart.

Stay Busy and Involved

As you head toward being a senior citizen, it's important that you stay busy and keep involved with your life. You can't allow yourself to slack off and do nothing with your days. This to me is the secret to growing older.

It's not good to sit around without something that can keep you alive and excited about the days ahead. Be more than a bump on a log!

At eighty-two, I can't see myself just relaxing or, as I call it, "collapsing." This isn't too good for your ambition and your desire to have something to do every day. Remember, if you become very lax in how you live your senior days, you will have nothing as the days move on. The body must be strong, the mind must be active. If you see the value of working on things that you can use later on, this is what is great about retiring or relaxing. (However you choose to call it.) To my mind, I think of how I can best utilize my hours and days.

If you stay busy and involved, you will keep from being bored. I talk myself into being occupied. Life is too short to waste time while developing your abilities. Staying busy is great. It's good for the mind. It motivates you to improve. Not keeping the mind involved every day is dangerous. The brain is complicated. I like to think that this is the secret of what life is all about. As far as I'm concerned, as we grow older the tendency is to allow ourselves not to get the most out of our talents.

At my present age of eighty-two, I see something in myself that makes my days wonderful. I've watched others get older and they somehow haven't been staying excited about advancing in their lives. For myself, I find I have become more enthusiastic as I have grown older.

Are You Able To Handle Being Alone As You Grow Older?

This has been a problem for many friends of mine these past many years. I see that keeping busy and joining clubs and other groups is important. Being alone can really keep your abilities and desires dulled. Not having something to do with our time can make us unhappy. Being happy in the senior years is very important. We must learn to keep a great frame of mind so we can make our senior days exciting and something to look forward to each day.

I am glad that I have something to do with my hours every day. This is what it's all about. We get up and ask ourselves what will we do Monday, Tuesday, Wednesday, Thursday, Friday, Saturday, and Sunday. We must have productive activities each day. We can't go to movies and shows and think this is sufficient to keep the brain alive.

I get up and know that I am still in beautiful physical condition, and this allows me to have the strength to practice my drums. I have something to write about with my study books and my literary ideas, and all of this makes it easy to look forward to each new day.

I like to look outside and say to myself, as the song says, "OH, WHAT A BEAUTIFUL MORNING, OH, WHAT A BEAUTIFUL DAY." The days in my life unfold and give me great pleasure just to be alive. Of course, I realize not all of us are fortunate enough to have some wonderful things to occupy our senior days. However, if we think back to when we were younger, maybe we'll see something in our past that can make the future brighter.

I don't know what to tell people, but I see for myself that I have a wonderful outlook and am doing something I love. I have never lost my love for music and my drum talents. Practicing and developing my abilities make my days just wonderful.

Now the desire to write my philosophy of life occupies my days. I spend a few hours a day at my typewriter and little by little my books about how I see life emerge. It's really amazing, because I never thought this could happen to me.

So I say, if this can happen to me at eighty-two, why can't it happen to others? Why shouldn't Jack, Joe, or Sally also have the drive to write and compose something about what they do, about what they love. Think about that, buddies. IT CAN HAPPEN.

If You Are Young, Have You Given Much Thought to How You Will Handle Growing Older?

Here's an interesting thought: When we are in our young adult years, do we give much thought to the days when we will reach our senior years? We know there aren't any guarantees about what we will do and how we will be prepared for our senior days. When we are young, this part of our life just doesn't seem important. We know in the back of our minds that this eventually will come about. We don't get younger, only older.

I have lived my young life and now I'm faced with my senior years. It's inevitable. It will happen to all of us. That is, if we are in good health and have the strength and abilities to carry on.

My suggestion to all is that we must have an idea about what we want to do when we get older. At what age do we wish to start preparing for our senior days? How will we handle our money? Will we have enough dollars to exist? Are the dollars we get from social security going to be enough for us and our family? Have we socked away the money to handle this stage of life?

Will we have to be TAKEN CARE OF BY OUR KIDS? WILL WE HAVE A PLACE TO LIVE, SLEEP, HANG OUR HAT, AND HAVE THE FOOD TO EXIST? There is so much we must think about. Many of us do not make adequate plans in our younger days. There is no question, my friends, if you haven't given it much thought, you'd better get on it.

I was so busy with being a professional musician that I didn't give my senior years much consideration. So what I am telling everyone is that we must keep these years in our head. It's going to happen and if you are not ready for it, well, look out, me buckos.

So while you are productive in your youth, think hard and work hard and, like the squirrels do, put those nuts away for your later years. You don't need a lot, but you'll have a reserve to depend on. It's a good feeling if you see it that way. Again I say, if you do this, you'll not be sorry. If you don't plan for your older years, you will be.

Are You Keeping Active As You Are Getting Older?

I am and I intend to stay active as long as I have all my "marbles." As long as my body is able and brain-computer can still function and process my thoughts, there's no reason why I shouldn't stay active.

I'm healthy and breathing pretty good and can see and hear and think; I'm going full-speed ahead. I always knew I would be capable of functioning on all cylinders, so I plan to continue on my path of doing what I love to do.

If you are approaching your senior years and have ideas as to what you wish to do with yourself as you grow older and can do your thing, go for it. You have read throughout my book that I was ALWAYS PLANNING TO BE IN GOOD FORM, NO MATTER HOW OLD I GOT. I always wrote and told people that Sam Ulano will be doing what comes naturally to him.

At my "young age," everything is working beautifully. I remain active with full confidence that I can do my practice and play and study and come up with ideas that make sense. There's no reason why this can't happen to you.

I've been asked when I plan to stop. Haven't I had enough of drumming, teaching, and studying? No, never have I ever felt I have "had it." I really don't see my being able to stop, dead cold. Maybe if or when I get ill and lose some of my abilities and think I have had it, then I might hang up my boxing gloves and say, "THAT'S IT!" I do not expect that to happen, not just yet. But as they always say, "NEVER SAY NEVER." We don't know and so we can't predict what is in store for us.

I've watched others sell their homes, move to Florida, and in a year or two come back from Florida saying they were unhappy and bored. Or, some of us move near our kids and the kids are unhappy that their parents moved near them and interfered with their lives. I don't want to live near my daughter in New Jersey or my son in California. They want to live their lives and I want to live mine. I always say I'm not ready for a nursing home. I'm not ready to have someone tell me how to enjoy my senior days. No sir!

If you are lucky to be alive and well and have an active mind, stick with it and get on with your life. The way I see it, I need space and I need fun in my older years and so staying active, working, and enjoying these years is what I find will make me a happy person on this earth. FUN, FUN, FUN.

Are You Going To Do All the Things You Wanted To Do As You Get Older?

Many of us have made plans about what we are going to do when we reach our senior years. "I'm going to fish and play in the sun," one of my buddies said. Another said, "I'm going to travel all over the United States. I'm going to buy a portable home and take the wife to see this great country of ours." Others have told me they would like to see all of Europe. Some said they loved golf and were going to be on the links every day. Some told me that they will just live in Florida, Arizona, maybe Canada, and just wanted to be left alone.

Sounds good to me, but it isn't the way I want to live my life out. Everyone has ideas about what they want to do. For me, I can't see giving up my beautiful lifestyle of music, drumming, playing, writing, listening to my Yankees, following other sports, and completing many of the projects I started some years ago. Now that I have the time, I want to "do my thing."

I can't see myself not developing and finishing ideas. Maybe I didn't have the bucks to complete what I liked, and now I see the way clear to be able to do the things that always made me happy and satisfied when I got them done. It took some hard work and a lot of keeping my nose to the grindstone.

I know when I was young, like lots of people my age, I thought I was going to conquer the world. I was going to be the best I could be and reap all the rewards by doing things I planned. Somehow I, like you perhaps, never did follow all these wonderful dreams. I then decided to put some of my ideas on the back burner, and my life went by, and many of my goals weren't completed. But somewhere along the way, I woke the sleeping giant in my brain and started to burn. The flames got bigger, and I saw a chance to fulfill my life's dreams. I decided to make my ideas come to life.

And you want to know something? Again I see my dreams coming true. I think this means I will do more of what I wish to do. It can be done if we just stick with it.

How Will You Occupy Twenty-four Hours a Day?

Many times my students and I get into philosophical discussions. One of our favorite topics is what to do with twenty-four hours a day.

Good topic. How will we occupy twenty-four hours every day? Will we have enough ideas to fill these hours? Will we still be doing some of the things as we get older that we have been doing while we still were young? We must realize that many changes will take place in our lives as we move on to being sixty, seventy, maybe eighty, and even further down the road. We can't just jump up as we reach our older years and, boom, there it is — something exciting that we love to do. We can't just pick it up and find it fills our hearts and minds, and life at that age becomes wonderful.

For myself, I knew I was still going to be working at my music and all of the things I was developing in my young days. "You're nuts," I was told. "Things will change and there is no way you could be doing as an older person what you were doing as a younger man. You'll see."

I would tell everyone, "If I have my health, I see no reason why I can't still be working at my first love. There is nothing else I would like to do as I grow old. All I have to do is stick to it, keep working at it, and as I get on in years, I am certain I will go full force ahead." No kidding, I was saying this way back "when," and here, writing this, I see that it can be done.

I know this may not work for all of us. I know heredity plays a big part in our lives, but I wonder if it has to be so. I know developing a strong body and a strong will to succeed and sticking with this plan can help. How much, I can't say, because I am not a medical man. But I have lived through a broken back, cancer, and now diabetes and still have a strong, healthy senior life. So I can occupy my wonderful senior years DAY BY DAY.

Are You Expecting Your Kids To Take Care of You?

This is interesting to me. Many people who have kids, when they get up there in age, find they may have to depend on their kids to help them exist or maintain their lives. There is no guarantee about this. We don't know how to think about this. For myself, I never planned to have my son and daughter take care of me, financially or otherwise. It sometimes is many years down the pike, so we just can't figure how things will develop in our older life.

I have always wanted to take care of myself. During all of my growing years I would say, "I'll take care of myself, and I will do my best to be able to handle this phase of my life." I liked my independence and couldn't see myself looking ahead to my children taking care of me and providing for me. I guess I am lucky because of how things worked out for me. At eighty-two, I am able to function and do okay by myself. I don't need a lot of dollars to live. I'm not a big eater. I don't have to have special meals, and I don't need to have expensive clothes and live "high off the hog" to exist.

I planned it this way because I like my privacy. Others may want to live near their children. I could do without that. I love my kids and grandchildren, but I still want my freedom.

There are many of us who feel our children "owe us" for what we did for them. The way I see it, your kids don't owe you a thing. Let them live and enjoy their lives without putting a burden on them. If your children love you and wish you to participate in their lives, all well and good, but don't expect that they must give you something in return for the fact that you are their parents. My Mom let her children fend for themselves. I agree with her.

Once my wife and I got married and left our homes, my Mom felt we were old enough to "do our thing." She was proud of all of her kids, but never expected anything more than us loving her. We had to love her because she was such a strong woman and showed us the way, but didn't make demands on any of us. She had all these children and handled everyone the same way, with no favorites. She loved us all. I think her way was the best; have your kids and, like flowers, let them grow.

For myself it was SO GREAT because I was allowed to develop my interests and no one interfered. No problems. Mom only expected respect from us and we had to respect others. She would say others would respect us in return.

Keep Your Weight Under Strict Control

A s you've been reading, you may have noticed that I put a great deal of emphasis on controlling weight and taking care of our physical life. Once again in this chapter I talk about controlling weight and the importance of working at keeping excess weight off our bodies.

One of the important parts of being a top professional is weight control. I always read that this ballplayer or that boxer is working on keeping his weight down. When I hear interviews or read about a professional athlete, there is always mention about keeping excess weight off their bodies. Too much weight slows them down, dulls their abilities and reflexes, and is detrimental to their success in their sport.

When I was up there at three hundred twenty pounds, I was so out of shape I really didn't know how bad I was. However, as I've said, I received a good education about to why one should watch his or her weight. It was hard at first but I eventually got the hang of it and convinced myself that I'd better take control. I did and I'm still working on my body.

I feel wonderful every time I sit down at my typewriter and write about weight problems. Once I made up my mind, I vowed never again to lose control of my weight. Along with my body conditioning program and controlling my weight, each day is beautiful, exciting . . . marvelous! All my systems are "go" as they say. My digestion is great, body parts all are working, full steam ahead. What can I tell you? It's just tremendous that I learned how and what to do to keep myself strong and ready for whatever may come my way.

When I ride the morning bus to my studio, I see many men and women in poor physical condition. They are fat, obese; just awful. I always want to tell these people that they are slowly but surely killing themselves. Yes, they are. I can't do anything about it because I don't think they would hear me and, besides, who am I to tell them?

I've told many of my overweight drum students that they are doing damage to their hearts, bodies, and minds, and they will pay the price later on. How do they say? "You can lead a horse to water, but cannot make him drink." TOUGH, I SAY. GET HOLD OF YOURSELF. YOU'LL LOVE YOURSELF IF YOU DO.

We Never Get Too Big To Stop Studying

Sometimes we think we know it all. This is dangerous. I have students studying with me for years. John Sarracco is now on his thirty-third year as a student of mine. Why would someone study thirty-three years with the same teacher? A student studies with someone who can put more into his or her life.

For example, so and so becomes the champion of the boxing world. Are you telling me that once they become champ they get rid of their trainers, their coaches, doctors, press people, managers, and all the people involved with bringing that person to the top of their career? No way. They need these people around them to keep their heads straight, to keep them in training, and to check them medically. All this goes into making them the champ.

I still study. I took lessons in writing, some harmony and theory and piano, and I study what other people do as they train. I may not take lessons formally from a drum teacher, but now that I have so many years as a percussion player, I am able to teach myself. I can read music, of course. I know how to stay in training and what I must do to stay on top as a professional. I know how to study. I know how to tell my students the way to train. I follow my own system of study as if someone else were teaching me.

It sounds strange, but I know how to teach others and how to teach myself. Yes, I can do that. There is a time in our lives when we become proficient in our chosen fields. By this time we know how to train and study and teach ourselves. I hope that makes sense to you.

We never are too great to study. I'm a big believer that we never should stop learning, no matter how old we get.

Study to me is like food. It is something that feeds us inside. It feeds the brain-computer. It tells us how to review, why we should review, and what we plan to gain from the hours we spend in our development. Study broadens our life. It gives us new perspectives. Study is the way to help our mind and body to grow. I call it "food for the brain." It's the food for our love of what we do.

Study makes us human and educated so we can go on to greater things in our lives. If this sounds like I am preaching to you, then so be it. When I study my craft I feel like I am being somebody. I feel as if I am reaching new heights in my goals that I can use in days to come. Study settles many things for me. I know where I am going, what I want to do with my life, and how I can get rewards in my life other than dollars.

Money is a tool. Study is food.

You Don't Need Heavy Weights

As I wrote throughout *I Love What I Do!* and here in *Keep Swinging!*, I emphasize staying in good physical shape and how we can do it with the help of free weights. These are not heavy weights, but weights that will be appropriate for most of us growing older. Ten, fifteen, twenty, and twenty-five pound weights will do the trick for you.

I think back to Sigmond Klein and his gym. It was on 48th Street and 7th Avenue, here in Manhattan. It was not a big gym, but it had most of the essential weights and benches that one would use in this type of training.

What was fascinating about Sigmond's system of free weights was that anybody could follow it. With his direction, one could really know what to do and how to do it. When I first started lifting weights, I started with a twenty-pound cross bar. I did ten lifts, bending over and straightening my body up. Remember, when I started I weighed three hundred twenty pounds and so I started slowly at first. I also used ten-pound barbells. Some called them dumbbells. I would try to lift the ten pounds over my head in a standing position. It was tough for me because I had never done this before.

After the first month of lifting these light weights, I started on bench presses. You lie down on a bench about two or three feet off the floor. In this position, I took a forty-pound cross bar and did what's called a "bench press." You are lying down, feet on the floor, looking up to the ceiling, pushing upwards. I would start with ten bench presses. This made my arms stronger and also was good for my back.

One thing to remember is that lifting weights doesn't mean we will lose weight from the lifting. We are just strengthening the muscles. To lose weight, one must watch what they eat, how they eat, and how much they eat. This was how I lost weight, week in and week out. After a year, I had dropped about eighty pounds and gained stronger arms, shoulders, legs, and torso. Together, controlling what I ate, cutting out some of my bad eating habits, lifting weights three and sometimes four days a week, I had it made! Having someone like Sigmond Klein directing me was the key, because I could follow his very strict routine. If I didn't, I would have been thrown out of his place. A NO-NONSENSE GUY. TOUGH, BUT GOOD-HEARTED.

Klein showed me that lifting light weights and sticking to the program works. It's now over forty-one years that I have stuck with this plan, watching what I eat, and how much I eat, and continuing my weight lifting program. It makes sense to me.

I even wrote a book entitled, *HOW TO LOSE WEIGHT AND FIT BEHIND YOUR WHEEL.* I don't drive any longer, but I can get behind the steering wheel. Thank God. I LEARNED TO LISTEN.

Never Stop

Before I was involved with my love for drumming and music, I really didn't have any reason to say to myself, NEVER STOP. I wasn't doing anything that I wanted to keep doing. My thoughts would wander all day and I would fantasize.

I'd think I was a cowboy or a doctor. Then I would be a fireman or a detective. I would never read a book, because I had NO INTEREST IN READING. As I wrote earlier, I was a horrible student. I really couldn't care less. Everyone in my family tried to tell me why I should study. They said if I didn't study I would suffer later on in my life. I couldn't understand that thought.

Subconsciously I knew my brothers and sisters were correct. My Mom also knew it was best that I learn to read and write, but she somehow would tell everyone that I eventually would get the hang of it and become a serious pupil. What she couldn't say, but she did feel inside, was that SAMMY would come around.

She would tell everyone to leave me alone. Eventually they did. When I started High School, during the first term, the music teacher spotted something about me that told him I was musically inclined. I had a special feeling for music. I was already playing drums and even taking lessons. He directed me to the principal's office to transfer me to the main building of James Monroe High School, on Boynton Avenue, in The Bronx.

We lived a half-block from the school. My first day in High School I was put into the band and orchestra. I loved it and loved the people who were in charge of these two groups. It was exciting and fun. Man, I was having a ball in school and this was the catalyst that set me off.

When I started to be interested in drums and music and I felt I had the ability to play this instrument, something came over me.

I was able to sit for hours and study and practice. I hadn't played my first job with a band, other than in school as yet. Mr. Firestein recommended me to a quartet that was playing various functions in and around The Bronx. My first encounter with a live band was to play with this quartet in a bar, for seven strippers. They took off all their clothes and promenaded up and down on this long bar. I didn't know what to do, so the band leader told me to play anything I wanted on my tom-toms.

I got home and told my Mother that these women were taking off their clothes. My Mom said, "Don't worry. You'll see a lot of that as you get older." I made two dollars, but because it was the Depression, two dollars was considered a lot of money. This band would have me play with them every week for almost a year. I really learned a great deal with these musicians. I always called it "ON THE JOB TRAINING," and it was.

This is why I tell my students to NEVER STOP because this gets you ready for whatever may come your way. NEVER STOP, NEVER GIVE UP. IT IS ONE OF THE KEYS TO SUCCESS.

Why Say You're Going To Do Something and Then Never Do It?

Promises, promises, promises. Broken promises. This is a terrible habit to have; saying you are going to do something and then not doing it. It's bad for your reputation in any field. People will lose their confidence in you and your abilities.

I know many people who do this. It's not a good policy and can turn others in your profession away from you and will affect how you are thought of in your business. I know of quite a few musicians who say they are going to record an album and never do it. Some even go so far as to put a band together, rehearse for weeks, and then the entire project falls apart. It's not healthy and can backfire on you if you are someone who does this. I know I wouldn't WANT TO BE INVOLVED WITH A PERSON WHO IS SO IRRESPONSIBLE.

My method of doing things is to plan what I want to do first, set aside the amount of dollars for expenses, talk it over with the musicians I am planning to use for their input about what they would like to see done and how they feel it should be done. I get some idea as to how much the musicians wish to be paid, and their ideas about the music and style of music we will record.

I recently put out an album; planned it out, the amount of studio time, how many tunes, and how I wanted to have them played. I set the dollars aside so I could pay the band after the session was completed. I got a signed agreement that I can promote and use the photos of each member in any form or manner I want to in order to advertise the recording.

There are lots of details when doing this type of thing in the music world and to have some credibility, I want every one in the band to know what's happening. I spell it all out for each member, following my concept of saying I want to do something and then doing it. No nonsense. Your fellow workers will respect you when your intentions are straightforward and you leave nothing to guesswork. **No indecision. No chance of saying I'm going right and then going left.**

I have learned that this is important both to me and to others. I am certain most of us will learn these lessons well as we advance to our senior years. The same thing has happened with my first book. The publishers approached me, I spelled out what would make me happy with our arrangements. They, in turn, did the same. Everything was written down on paper. We both agreed what would be to each of our advantages and we signed on the dotted line. Everything up front. No questions left unanswered. It's the same principle if you buy a house or a car, where there are papers to sign and you agree that you are going to do something. **Do it.**

Confidence and Conceit

There are two interesting words about which many of us eventually learn. My good friend Buddy Rich had always been labeled as a very conceited A-HOLE. He would say to me that most people don't know the difference between these two words: CONFIDENCE IS WHEN YOU KNOW YOUR THING, CONCEIT IS WHEN YOU THINK YOU KNOW YOUR THING.

Buddy would say to me, I KNOW WHAT I AM DOING and I am CONFIDENT THAT I AM DOING IT TO THE FULLEST OF MY ABILITIES. He always said he didn't have to be conceited because he was very sure of himself. One of the problems, he would say, is that people thought he was conceited.

I guess all of us, when we are young, might be conceited. We really don't know our abilities and so conceit comes through in our personality. Once we know what we are doing there is no need to act conceited to cover up the fact that we don't know our craft.

I can honestly say that I was probably very conceited in my early years. I was a big blowhard and had to learn the hard way until I reached a point in my life where I became confident about my talent. I most likely was an I/ME KIND OF CAT. "I" this, and "Me" that, and "I", "I," "I" and "Me," "Me," "Me" — and so forth. Eventually I learned this was not the way to be. I got my conceit under control.

I stopped being an "I"/"Me" kind of person and let my talent do the talking. Blustering and boasting stopped being a part of my makeup. SHUT YOUR MOUTH, SAM ULANO. I noticed this worked pretty well for me. It became my motto. Only speak when spoken to and only speak when I know what I am talking about. So everyone who goes through the conceited front eventually gets the message about being only a confident person.

As I grew up and eventually knew what I was talking about and what I was doing and what my industry was about, I lost my conceit and swagger and found myself being just me. I learned my lesson well. It's unfortunate but my educators never stopped me from being such a conceited ass. I wish they had. It could have saved me lots of problems as a working player.

BUDDY RICH said it so well. A great statement by one of the music giants of all times. I loved that man. I respected his abilities and what he had to say to his fellow musicians. Too bad many took him to be a conceited jerk. He wasn't. He was a great human being. Many of us learned from him. Thank God I was smart enough to listen.

Have You Decided What Will Happen to Your Life's Work "After You've Gone?"

A s the song says, "AFTER YOU'VE GONE . . ." What thoughts have you given to this aspect of your life? We must give this some serious thinking. I know I have to think of what I want done with my large collection of writing, videos, audio tapes, literary work about my methods of teaching and playing. I am certain many of us have created a body of work, not only in the music field but in all fields of endeavor.

Some of us die off and never have made arrangements. My son and I have discussed what is going to happen to all the material I have created. It's a serious part of this life of ours. We can't just let everything hang in midair.

At eighty-two, I have given much thought to this. I really haven't figured it all out yet, but I am now in the process of writing and spelling out what I want done. My son and daughter will be in charge of this tremendous gathering of books and other ideas I have documented over these years of my life.

My philosophy of life enters into this phase of what I'd like to see done with everything. Some of my books I have left to John Sarracco, a student who has been like a second son to me all of these years. He is progressive enough to know what to do with what I have assigned to him. Bill Rotella in Waterbury, Connecticut, also will share in what I leave over. It's not dollars and cents, but Bill, like John Sarracco, knows what to do with this kind of material. At this point I am not ready to pass on. But one never knows what will be, so we must spell it out.

I have given consideration to donating some of my work to the PERCUSSIVE ARTS SOCIETY. They have a library of material that creators like myself can send items. These materials will stay alive in their care. That's what they are about. It's sort of a museum. They look after the MATERIAL THAT PEOPLE IN OUR INDUSTRY CREATE.

There are other options and ways that we can seek to perpetuate our life's work. We just have to document it. Part of the purpose of my Philosophy of Life at eighty-two is to make people aware that they must think about this. Some people donate parts of their bodies to the medical profession. Some donate money to colleges and other serious places in this wonderful world of ours. You just have to know how to spell it out in simple and clear language. Think. Make a decision as to just what you want to happen to the creative part of your life. I think we all must take stock of this. DECIDE WHAT TO DO NOW, BECAUSE YOU CAN'T, "AFTER YOU'VE GONE."

Have a Typewriter Handy So You Can Type Your Ideas Out

I've found this to be a good suggestion: Have a typewriter close by in case you have thoughts that you would like to put on paper right away. Here I am at the ripe old age of eighty-two and I have two typewriters on hand, because I like to get my thoughts down on paper. Who knows what I'll write out with a machine ready for whatever my mind might conjure up.

My typewriter gets quite a workout.

Every day I write for about a half-hour and sometimes more. To me, typing is so much better than writing by hand. Over these many years I have had the opportunity to do some serious writing with my typewriter. I might suggest the Brother-79 typewriter. This machine is not too expensive.

At night, I write out topics that I want to cover. I type a few pages every day. This system is so great for me. It allows me to get my thoughts ready for whenever I have the time to type. I never say to myself that I am too busy and haven't got the time to write. I make the time. I must make the time because ideas come and go. *My Book of Philosophy at Eighty* was completed in a very short time. The same with this book. I eventually get to all the topics and then am ready to have my editor take care of the details of correcting a lot of the errors I make in punctuation and grammar.

You people out there who have ideas and procrastinate in getting them down on paper make a sad mistake. Put your typewriter to work. No one else will do this for you.

I find typing like talking to myself. I ask myself questions and even answer the question for myself. In fact, it is sort of crazy. If some people heard me talking to myself, they would say that I am on the wacky side. I guess I am a bit loco, but who cares? I know it and I don't care who else knows it.

However, that is the least important part of all of this. I type, love to type, and eventually get my ideas down on paper. *I LOVE WHAT I DO!* was very rewarding for me. I wrote it as a hobby with no thought of having it published. And here is Book Two. It's just super that this happened. Who knows? I may eventually do a Book Three. Good things have happened because my handy, dandy typing machine was ready.

Give this idea some serious thought. It's like having food in your fridge for when you might want a quick snack. Open the fridge and, bango, you are set. My typewriter helps to store the food of my brain. Look at it as if you want to talk to yourself and your machine takes dictation. Great fun.

As They Say in Lotto, You Never Know

I don't know how it works outside of the BIG APPLE, but here in New York we have a saying, "YOU CAN'T WIN IT IF YOU ARE NOT IN IT." I have sort of proven this to myself. I wrote *MY PHILOSOPHY OF LIFE AT EIGHTY* for fun and now it's published in a beautiful form. You never know.

It's like someone writes a hit song and has to wait until it is recorded and played on the radio and then gets on the charts and sells millions of copies. YOU NEVER KNOW. I was talking to a friend of mine who wrote a collection of poems. He put the collection back in his dresser drawer and for many years it stayed there. We got to talking and he found my "pearls of wisdom" very exciting. He tells me he is going to take the collection of poems and rewrite them and maybe get inspired to get them published. I told him, "HEY, RAY, YOU NEVER KNOW."

I've asked many friends if they've ever written anything that had some potential. Good question. We, as part of the average public, don't know what value something we did may have. HOW COULD WE KNOW? THERE IS NO WAY WE WOULD KNOW, UNLESS WE WERE IN THE BUSINESS.

Many years ago, I heard MITCH MILLER, who was able to discover many singing artists and helped produce hit records for them. I heard him on a radio talk show. He was asked how come he was able to produce so many hit singles and LPs. He answered that IF HE KNEW, HE WOULD BE A GENIUS. He explained to the audience that there was a great deal of luck in his business and this luck caused things to happen.

I have asked a few people if they believe in luck. They said they did, but couldn't explain it. It just happens like a flash of lightning. YOU NEVER KNOW. But if I hadn't made this collection of notations about what I wanted to write, I would never have had a chapter ready in the YOU NEVER KNOW category that became a part of this beautiful book.

If You Wanted To Go from New York City to Los Angeles, You'd Get a Map!

This is one of my favorite concepts: about not knowing how to go from New York to Los Angeles and what to do about that. You'd get a map and this map would tell you how to travel from Point A to Point B. I think that's very simple. It's easy. This is a logical way to think.

Over all my years, I knew this was a very good way to understand what to do and how to do it. GET A MAP.

When I don't know something I get a map or I look up the literature about a subject and I research it. We eventually get smarter and understand. We have to check our brain and see what we have stored that could help us know what to do.

As we grow up to know our capabilities, we start to see things more clearly. It sounds simple and maybe it is, but through some experience of understanding ourselves, the answers show up. I am surprised at myself. I went from being a complete dummy in my early years and (without bragging), I find my mind and thinking processes got so much better. Why? I guess I finally learned how to use my brain and the ideas I had stored up there.

I always say there must be a way to do what we want to do. There is always a way to learn what we want to learn. As the song says, "THERE MUST BE A WAY," and I am convinced if we study, learn, develop our abilities, there must be a way to answer what needs to be answered. It can be done.The hunt and search using the map is what fascinates me. I'm sure you too will find this hunt and discovery a fascinating way to find the method of doing what you want to do.

The trick is getting that map. Trial and error. Review and study. Work at developing your mind to reveal what you are seeking. Once you find the secret, you then will reap the rewards of the hunt. Great, isn't it?

Find Out What You Do Best and Then
Train Your Brain in Your Strong Points

I think this makes a lot of sense. TRAIN YOURSELF IN YOUR STRONG POINTS; WHAT YOU THINK YOU ARE BEST IN IS WHERE YOU WANT TO CONTRIBUTE YOUR HOURS. That's what I did. My philosophy in life was to know what my best talent was and what I love to do. I studied my feelings very seriously, and when I came to the conclusion that I loved drumming and the music world so much, then this was where my drive should be.

I gave it my best shot. I talked to myself and asked myself if I was interested in spending the many hours necessary to develop my skills as a professional player. I came up with the answer that I was talented enough to be a good, solid drummer. I also knew I had the abilities to teach others and discovered that teaching was also one of my desires. I was able to look down the pike and knew that Sam Ulano could be a capable drummer. I didn't think I would be the only person who could be a class act at the drum set, however.

How did I know? It was more a feeling that I could be what I wanted to be. It wasn't easy. I had to give up a lot of things in my life that others wouldn't, but I said to myself that I could see myself spending my whole life doing what I love to do.

How can someone find out what they do best? How can they know what they will love to do all their lives? There is no method that can answer this question for us. Trial and error is the way I found out. In my mind, there is no way to know for sure, but I do think we can feel something about ourselves. I just knew in my heart and mind that I was on the right track.

I would get up every day and feel something stirring inside of me. I just knew: DRUMS, DRUMMING, AND EVERYTHING CONNECTED WITH THAT BURNING DESIRE INSIDE OF ME. THAT WAS HOW I KNEW.

I still can't put my finger on what was happening to me. But what a wonderful life I have had in music. It has made me so happy.

I can't get into someone else's mind and heart, but I feel I am no different than the next person. To me, I think we all can feel strongly about what we want from ourselves. I do think we all have these sensitivities.

YOU MUST BE THE JUDGE. YOU HAVE TO SEARCH WITHIN YOURSELF TO FIND JUST WHAT YOU WOULD LOVE. I did it and still am doing it. I must now stick with it. This is my answer and this is how I will follow my path to a successful life. **I REALLY LOVE WHAT I DO.** And I guess I always will.

Remember, Your Brain Is the Storeroom for Your Thoughts

C an you picture this? You have a couple of special rooms in your home or apartment, where you may store extra furniture or use for extra books. Maybe you make it your musical practice room. Or perhaps you can store your computer in this room, make it your guest room, or make it an extra bedroom.

I look at my brain as this extra room where I store my ideas. Now mind you, I don't really use my brain to store everything. Sometimes I write my ideas down. My accumulated life's work lives in my brain. I call on my brain to tell me what I can do with my drum talents, how to solo, or how to write a new percussion book. I call my brain the place I store my nuts, like a squirrel.

My brain has a switch that I can turn on or off. I turn the switch on when I am awake and turn it off when I want to go to sleep or rest. Ideas are stored up and lay dormant until I have that desire to use them.

In all my years I never fully appreciated the value of my brain. However, as I advanced in my life, I came to see where I and many of us never made full use of this wonderful part of our body. Yes, eyes, ears, nose, private parts, stomach, heart, and so forth — these parts of our body are important. We must keep them "oiled" and in the best shape possible. BUT THE BRAIN, what a marvelous invention of our Creator, to give each of us our own unit! Every one of us gets this unique mechanism. Each of us has our own private brain. We take it to sleep with us every night. We travel with it wherever we go.

This great machine comes with its own carrying case. This wonderful part of the body controls everything we do. It's so private and it is such a grand item. We don't need MICROSOFT, IBM, OR AT&T, OR ANY OTHER COMPANIES TO GET PARTS FOR US. We store all of our information and when we want the information it appears on its own screen in the carrying case. Isn't that great? I love the fact that I woke my brain up this morning and it is now ready for whatever use I wish.

Feed Things into Your Brain

Feeding our brain is like feeding our stomachs. We put food into our bodies to give us energy. It's like gasoline that runs our car. We feed ideas into our brain and that gets our mind and body going.

You must find a way to store ideas in your brain. Then when you want some ideas, there they are! This is what I built my philosophy of life upon. I eventually got to a point where my computer brain spit it all out and of course, my philosophy books took shape and form.

When I was very young, my family tried to convince me that I needed to study and learn. I didn't want to be bothered with study. I look back now and I see that I suffered as a young person. I didn't die and I wasn't punished by anyone, but I think I would have done better as a young man if I had put the effort into adding to my brain. I look back now and realize that I was stupid.

I once read a book about how to study and the writer said that many of us only use about two percent of our brain power. He went on to say how much better we would be if we used even ten to twenty percent of our brain power. I think back on that statement and totally agree with him. Who knows? I might have been a genius!

In the classic film, THE WIZARD OF OZ, the TIN MAN wanted to have a heart, the LION wanted to have courage, the STRAW MAN wanted a BRAIN. Each wanted something special. THE WIZARD OF OZ showed each of them that they already had what they wished for and how best to use it.

We have the brain, and now, we must develop and use it. It's unfortunate that I didn't learn this in my early years, but I had to mature to come to this realization. But it's really so simple, isn't it?

Train Your Brain

Train your brain every day, one-half hour or an hour a day or devote whatever free time you can to developing your brain.

My philosophy of life seems to talk a lot about health and our brain power. I keep thinking a great deal about these two aspects of living. Why this has been happening to me in these later years of my life, I can't say, but in the back of my mind these topics seem to take priority. In my drum teaching I stress these two topics to my students. When they read from a drum instruction study book, I try to impress upon them that their body doesn't think. It's their mind that helps them see what they want to play. Only by using their brain can they develop their ability. Only by transporting ideas into the "machine" that sits on top of their shoulders.

To me that makes sense, because in my early days as a beginning student, I was very involved in physical playing and not mental playing. This happens to all students of music. WE THINK THE PHYSICAL ACTION IS MOST IMPORTANT. It is not. It has nothing to do with how well we can perform. WE MUST THINK.

I have learned that only my brain can direct me. Nothing else. Of course, the other topic I write a great deal about is taking care of our health and bodies. Even here we must use our brains and learn as much as we can about what to do and what not to do to keep ourselves in the best of health. We don't have to be a fanatic about our health, but we must get educated to know what makes our bodies "tick." That way we can perform at our very best.

Eventually, as we grow older, we understand ourselves and how our brain works. I have learned that I never will reach my goals and realize my ambitions if I don't work from my computer brain, and I am so happy that I have learned this.

Work at this and someday your ideas will pop out and you will have all these ideas at your fingertips. It works for me and it may just work for you. Give it a chance to develop.

What Would Keep You Happy in Your Senior Years?

I guess I am always talking about being happy in our older years. I think it's great if we find something that can keep us enjoying our life. By now most of you who have read my first book know that Sam Ulano has found the secret of happiness.

Keep in mind that hunting for a method of staying on top of your health to me is uppermost. If you are young and reading what I have to say, it might set you off in the right direction regarding how you can stay in good condition until you are a senior. As you reach your senior days, good health may be the secret of building happiness.

I always think about PONCE DeLEON, who set out to find the fountain of youth. Eventually he realized this place was actually in his mind. I agree with that. Staying in excellent health can lead you to this place in your mind. I call it THE BUILT-IN FOUNTAIN OF YOUTH, and we have been carrying it within our minds all of our lives. If you can discover this wonderful life in your brain, you've got it made.

We all mature and how we conceive of this aging process is a big part of our development. The way I see it, once I know in my mind that this fountain of youth is within me, I can then find THE WORLD OF HAPPINESS. When I decide what makes me happy I have a good idea about how I will live my senior years.

What a great sensation it is to find what makes us happy. This can give us the drive to improve. This can give us something to look forward to each waking day of our lives. To get up in the morning and have something we love to do keeps us happy. That "something" that makes life a joy. And it might give us the drive to accomplish something with the years, other than spending our time waiting for our social security check. The great fun of having some special thing to do, is that, who knows, we might even make a small living from it.

I don't know too many seniors who are still productive. Many are not happy and this isn't fun. YOU HAVE TO SEARCH YOUR HEART AND MIND. THEN YOU'LL FIND WHAT WORKS FOR YOU.

What Are You Expecting from Others?

This is a thought that runs through my mind every so often. What do we really expect from other people? Do they owe us anything? Do we depend on them only because they are our friends? My philosophy of life has brought me to this conclusion: I EXPECT THE SAME THING FROM OTHERS THAT I EXPECT FROM MYSELF. That's the way I see it.

I've written that no one owes me anything and so it fits together with this idea. I feel that I am not looking for anything special from others. They have nothing to give me. I have nice friends and I don't impose any demands on these friends. I just enjoy them as my friends. I don't try to ask them for money, I don't try to have them "pull my chestnuts out of the fire." I just love them all for who they are, and we enjoy each other's lives without demands.

There is nothing that they can give me that I need. At Christmas, we send each other season's greetings. We wish each other happiness when the years change, and we sort of remember each other's birthdays. Sometimes they invite me to their home for Thanksgiving or Easter or we just go out and enjoy supper or hear a band every so often.

What can we expect from each other? I don't want to be friends with someone who wants to borrow dollars from me. This turns me off. I don't want to be friends with people who depend on me all the time and want to occupy my hours more than just a short "hello" and good wishes. Others have a life, I have a life. I need my space and I am certain that we all need breathing space.

What else should we expect from people we know? From family? From relatives? I don't want to impose my problems on others. No one should take up our time telling us all their troubles. I tell people to get a doctor that can help them with worries. I don't expect others to shoulder my difficulties. It would be an imposition on others and on myself.

I cite the case of a dear friend who wanted me to co-sign a fifty-thousand-dollar note because he was in debt and deep trouble. He hadn't talked to me for ten years and eventually got in touch with me and we sort of made up. It was never the same. Inevitably, we drifted apart. He had been one of my closest friends. However, this demand he made on me to sign papers to help him get this loan ruptured our relationship. So you see, my philosophy has taught me, be my friend, but don't expect me to live your life. I have my own to live and that's all I want.

Control Your Food Intake

Consistently running through the books of my philosophy of life is the theme of the importance of taking control of our body, our health, and always being on top of our physical development. I once again stress this subject. It is of uppermost importance in my life and I constantly want to highlight this to you and explain why it is so important.

I talk about a system of exercise. A great deal of how well we will be and how well we will feel every day depends on this. You must realize this, and the sooner you do, the better off you'll be.

A significant part of staying in good health is how and what we eat. I am not a nutritionist and I am not a medical doctor. I can only tell you how I attacked this problem. As I told you, I was up to three hundred twenty pounds. I was FAT, SLOPPY, OUT OF SHAPE, OBESE, wearing a size fifty-four jacket, a size fifty-two waistline, and a size eighteen shirt! I was just a physical wreck. This was when I realized that I was a mess. What can I tell you? As my dear friend SIGMOND KLEIN said when he met me, (and please excuse my language but it's the only way I can tell you what he said to me), "SAM, YOU ARE ONE HUNK OF FAT SHIT." That's what he said to me.

I said to him, "WHAT ARE WE GOING TO DO ABOUT IT?" And he shot back at me, "WHAT ARE WE GOING TO DO ABOUT IT? SAM, WHAT ARE YOU GOING TO DO ABOUT IT? I don't have to do a thing. That is your problem." Sigmond then added, "HOW LONG DID IT TAKE FOR YOU TO GET INTO THIS CONDITION?" I told him it was about twenty-five years. Klein said, "Well, it's going to take you twenty-five years to undo your problem of being overweight."

So it went. And it made so much sense to me. We got started on our program of body conditioning. Now Klein said to me, "You have to find a better way to eat. Control your food intake. Eat what you like," he told me, "but, cut back on a lot of things." I made a list of what I was eating and followed this program.

I cut out bread, butter, dairy foods like cheese, eggs, cream cheese; mayonnaise, fried foods and discontinued eating before bedtime. I made my evening food intake at seven o'clock. I cut everything down and stuck with this program of eating. No pizza, no hot dogs, very little meat, chicken, fish. I eat everything but cut the size of my portions. I cut out cakes, chocolate, candies, ice cream. In fact, I cut down on everything "I loved." And I have stayed with that until this day. AMEN.

If You Have To Be Somewhere
at a Certain Time,
Try To Be There
a Little Ahead of Time

My motto has always been to leave yourself some extra time when you have to be someplace. This applies to a "gig" or an appointment with a doctor, an interview, whatever it may be. Always try to get there slightly early. It pays to think this way. If you are driving or going by train; if you have to catch a plane, allow yourselves some extra space. This will allow you to be relaxed and cut down on the pressure that comes with not being on time.

This has worked all of my life. Get there early and you'll never be late. Now at the age of eighty-two, I can talk from experience. I never know what is happening on the road if I drive. I don't really know what the weather conditions are. It could rain and thunder. There could be a serious accident on the road. I say we never know. In fact, there is no way to know. If you are flying somewhere, always get to the airport early to check your baggage, check in, and be ready to board the plane with time to spare.

If you are traveling by train or bus, again I say, leave plenty of time to get there. I always leave lots of time so I can have a cup of coffee and read my paper and be cool, so I don't get frustrated and aggravate my tummy. I want to be ready at all times.

Map out your plans. If you are taking clothes, have your luggage packed and ready to go. Sometimes it pays to ship your baggage ahead of you, maybe two or three days before you travel. If you play drums and must take your instrument with you, get it ready and packed so it can be handled with time to spare. My version of the old Boy Scout motto is: **"BE READY, JUST IN CASE."**

I'm a total fanatic when I have to be somewhere and want to make sure I'm there on time. I get all my things together and can handle the situation as it comes up. I'm not a fortune-teller and I can't predict the future, but I can be ready for it. My many years have taught me this concept. My philosophy of life tells me that this works all the time. Leave no loose ends.

I make a list as to what has to travel with me. It usually includes my cameras, film, extra batteries, maybe some of my books for display, and my drum sticks, just in case I'm called upon to play. I want to make sure I have the things I can control under full control.

I think it's a good habit to develop. The song says, "Straighten Up and Fly Right." I say, to fly right, we must make our minds ready for the trip. So take it from old man Sam, always be ready and you'll have the situation covered. You can't miss.

Don't Sell Yourself Short

Many of us have a habit of playing ourselves down. We get to thinking that if we show we are sure of ourselves, people will get an idea that we are being overbearing and "coming on strong." I don't feel that way. I don't feel I'm cocksure of myself and come on strong. I think it's good to feel we know our stuff.

I know what I can do and don't see any reason to play myself down . . . I'm very sure of myself and I think it's good. For me, it's healthy and I really don't care how others view me.

I've spent sixty-nine years in my craft. I have practiced my "tush" off, as the saying goes. I really "paid my dues," the hard way, every day of my growing life. I have learned my skills when it comes to playing my instrument. Yes, I know there are areas of the music world that I have not nailed down yet, but there is time in my life to develop those parts that I still need to work on. I'll eventually get the hang of it and be able to perform in those areas of MUSIC as well.

However, right now I can do about ninety percent of my work. This is my opinion of what I can do and I don't sell myself short. I think it's bad to make it look like I'm not sure of how well I can do my thing in my field.

You will learn to be sure of yourself in your chosen field if you have studied, trained, and still are staying on top of your abilities. I say if others get the idea that I am too sure of myself, well, that's too bad. It's healthy to be certain of yourself.

I think that if, after all these years, I gave people the feeling that I'm not sure of myself, then I will suffer. I will not be called for work, because those who want to use my talents might hesitate if I showed this lack of certainty about my abilities.

I have watched most of the top pros in my field. When they are on stage, they know what they are doing and can do it as a top professional. I'm talking about Sinatra, Ella, Benny, Artie Shaw, Harry James, Louis Armstrong, to name a few. In baseball, the top players know they can hit, run, catch the ball, and play their game. In football, in boxing, basketball — no matter what area of life — those who can do, can do. Those who can't do have and give a feeling that they are not certain. **THE PROFESSIONAL NEVER SELLS HIMSELF SHORT.**

You see it in their eyes and manner, the way they carry themselves, and how they talk about themselves. There is a feeling that they are sure and certain about who they are and what they can produce. I feel the same way.

In America, Everyone Has a Chance

In this marvelous country of ours we all have a chance to do something with our lives. Of course that is if we want to do something with ourselves. This doesn't mean we all will be famous. What I am saying is that we all can strive to be the best we can be. We must decide what we want, and then the hard work must start. This way we can go after what we want to do with our lives.

As I wrote in *I Love What I Do!*, I believe that had I been in any other country than America, I wouldn't have done the things I wanted to do and did do. I recall corresponding with a drummer in Czechoslovakia, some years ago. He and I were "pen pals," so to speak. I'd get a letter from him maybe once a month and I would answer him. We would exchange audio tapes in which he would ask some questions. I would send an audio tape back to him with the best answers that I could give.

Well, as the years went on, I got a letter from this drummer friend saying he was not allowed to write to me any longer. He couldn't buy some of my books, he couldn't send money out of his country. He was restricted to a point where we finally lost track of each other. His last letter told me he wrote a drum instruction book and he was not allowed to publish it or send it to me even in its basic, unprinted form.

I thought that was terrible and it made me feel sad. However, I knew that only in **America** can we have the freedom to say what we like to say, be who we want to be, think as we would like to think. I'm certain we all know what this gentleman was saying to me. How lucky we are. As long as we don't disrupt other peoples' lives, as long as Sam Ulano doesn't bother you, he can do his thing.

No one stops us from doing this. No one says we have to buy this book or that book. It's our dollars to spend as we wish. My publisher, Vital Health Publishing/**ENHANCEMENT BOOKS** in Danbury, Connecticut, felt my book was worth the effort to put on the literary market and so they did.

ONLY IN AMERICA. I guess there are other places where it's possible to write and have your written word published, but I feel there is more of an opportunity to do this here. It is wonderful and a grand feeling that in this country we can be somebody and no one says we can't. If you want to become president, the governor, the mayor, a lawyer, a doctor, a scientist, whatever your heart's desire is, if you work at it and study, you can be who you want to be. Isn't that great? I say it is and thank God that it is so. "Thank you, **GOD.**"

You Must Have the Goods

When I was a young fellow getting involved with drums, my relatives would visit the house and say to my Mom, "Jenny (my Mother's name) if Sammy WOULD ONLY GET A BREAK." My Mother would answer them with her favorite remark, "WHEN SAMMY GETS THE GOODS, HE WILL GET THE BREAKS."

This always stuck in my mind . . . "IF SAMMY GETS THE GOODS, HE WILL GET THE BREAKS." Mom was right. YOU HAVE TO HAVE THE GOODS. If you don't have the goods, you can't make it. Actually, Mom was saying that you had to know your business. You had to be outstanding in your field and this was the "goods." Having the goods, you were able to compete in this wide world, no matter what your field.

I used to sit in my practice room and tell myself every day over and over again, "SAMMY WILL GET THE GOODS." I WOULD REPEAT THIS OVER AND OVER EVERY DAY OF MY GROWING LIFE. IN FACT, I MADE A POSTER OF MYSELF DRUMMING AND IT SAID, "Sammy Gets the Goods." You know what? I am certain I got the goods!

In fact, I am getting more of the goods every living day of my life.

It's interesting as I write this part of my philosophy of life, from deep in my subconscious mind, all these things from my early life are coming back to me. I just told my lady friend, Michele, that it's like writing a confession of my life. Everything is flashing up like a computer screen and my hands just type it out. I looked up and this was page one hundred one and I haven't even put a dent in what I want to write.

To those of you who are reading my thoughts about my life, you might find this could set you off and maybe you too could document your inner thoughts about your life.

MOM WAS SO RIGHT, SAMMY HAS TO HAVE THE GOODS TO GET TO WHERE HE WANTS TO BE IN HIS LIFE. I look back to the time when my Mother made this very profound statement and realize how true this was. I would hear my aunts and uncles discussing how a young person might reach their goals. My aunts would say that I had to know somebody who would take me under their wing, so to speak.

My aunts and uncles would discuss this with my Mother and tell her that someone has to give me the break. Mom would say again and again, **"WHEN SAMMY GETS THE GOODS, HE WILL MAKE HIS OWN BREAKS."** My aunts and uncles didn't believe this, but my Mom stuck to this idea. She was so certain. I agree, because my life has proven her right after all these years. **NO ONE DID IT FOR ME.**

Give Yourself a Chance

We must learn something as we grow. WE MUST GIVE OURSELVES A CHANCE TO USE OUR TALENTS. We can't be afraid to give ourselves a chance. We might create something special. We must give our talent a chance to grow and be exposed to the world.

I know it's not easy. I know there may be a subconscious feeling in the back of our minds that our talent is not what others want and so we don't take the opportunities that come. We are frightened or worried that nothing will happen for us. So we put our talent aside. We don't give ourselves a fair chance. We have come to a fast conclusion that what we created or what we can do will not be considered important in this sometimes pessimistic world of ours.

My motto is: GIVE YOURSELF A CHANCE. If it fails, so what? If it is scary to you that your invention, book, film idea, or whatever it is you have just isn't good enough for the world, you judge yourself too harshly and that's the end of your chance for success.

I tell you the truth, if I felt that way, *I LOVE WHAT I DO: A DRUMMER'S PHILOSOPHY OF LIFE AT EIGHTY* would never have developed as it has. If I thought that no one would like what I did, no one would like to read it, no one would ever notice my work, IF I THOUGHT THAT WAY, NOTHING WOULD HAVE HAPPENED.

Honestly, I never ever had negative thoughts like that. I can't be a coward about showing my work to people. I GIVE MYSELF A CHANCE. I always think this way: "HEY, LOOK WHAT I HAVE DONE. WHAT DO YOU THINK OF IT?" Well, I'll tell you, almost everyone I know has been sincerely supportive of my writing.

No one said, "it stinks." No one put it or me down. I'm talking about many friends, family, students, educators, the entire group of people who read it. No one thought that I was cracked in the

194

head. "Hey, Sam, GO FOR IT." I wrote it out of fun and my feelings for people. I gave myself a chance with no hesitation. I say this: If you don't give yourself a chance, you'll never know what you are able to accomplish in your life. I call this positive thinking. Now at eighty-two, I think I am starting a new part of my life. GIVE YOURSELF A CHANCE AND SEE WHAT HAPPENS. It's worth the effort.

English and Math to Me Are the Two Most Important Subjects We Must Study in America

Many years ago I was having a discussion with friends and we were asking the question, WHAT ARE THE TWO MOST IMPORTANT SUBJECTS THAT WE SHOULD STUDY IN AMERICA? I said I thought that ENGLISH and MATH were the two main studies we should try to master, if we can.

If you think of it, you too will come to the same conclusion that I did. Without these two studies you will find yourself very limited in this wonderful land.

Of course, we need ENGLISH so we can communicate. To talk, to read, and WRITE ENGLISH to me is so important. We would be at a loss if we couldn't read and write ENGLISH. It would be a problem. In fact, I told my buddies that if I were running the Board of Education, English and Mathematics would be the two major subjects I would want the students to learn. Other subjects are secondary to me.

I know we should learn as much as possible so we can broaden our knowledge. However, to me, first and foremost WE NEED ENGLISH and MATH. When I was young, I wished I was better at ENGLISH and MATH. As I matured, I woke up and took care of business and made a great deal of progress in my understanding of these two subjects.

Math is so important in reading drum music as well as in all phases of music. I'm certain you might have seen my mention of math and music in the first book of my philosophy of life. I say that once I was alerted to the importance of math in the study of music, I made great strides in learning math and was able to make use of it in writing my drum studies.

I've told you that as I got older and started to write my philoso-phy of life, all of these flashbacks made me aware of what my life was about. Now that I'm sort of documenting my thoughts, I can tell you that these ideas have become so much clearer to me. I tell it to you so you can also wake up to the importance of all of this as we advance in our lives.

Everyone in my family finally knew that I had "arrived," now that I was able to write my thoughts about life. I use a great deal of this in my drum instruction with my pupils. I try my best to wake them up not only about learning how to play the instru-ment but how to live life and become a "MENSCH." (YIDDISH for being a PERSON.)

"It's Not What You Know,
But Who You Know." Total Bull!

It's a very famous line. I've heard it for so many years. "IT'S
WHO WE ARE AND NOT WHAT WE KNOW" THAT WAS MOST
IMPORTANT TO BEING SUCCESSFUL. I say that is a total crock of
garbage. NONSENSE. Yes, sometimes knowing the right people
helps us get ahead, but you must know your craft and must be
able to produce. You can know a great many influential people in
your field, but if you are not trained and can't handle the job at a
top level, no one needs you.

There are people who have succeeded in their lives because of
contacts and the people they know in high levels who can give
them a push. That's nice, but you can't be in that top position
without being ready for the gig. In music, if you expect to play
with the best, you have to be one of the best. It's been proven over
and over. I have seen this happen time and time again.

Someone arrives on the scene and "makes it," so to speak, but
never has the ability to follow up. It's always, "What happened to
so and so?" So who you know doesn't always fly. It's great to have
the ability to know Mr. Jones or Mrs. Jones and use these connec-
tions but don't tell me you don't have to know your abilities to get
to what you want in your field. You must know and be able to
produce. You can't make it only on lip service.

Again I remind you of what my Mom always said: "You have to
have the goods." Even in today's times, I still say who you know
is nice, but what you know is better. This is how I see it.

I like the satisfaction of knowing I did it on my own merit. I did
it on my abilities and all of the hard study and work contributed
to my success. I got here on my own. If, after I make it and outside forces help me, like Vital Health Publishing/ENHANCEMENT
BOOKS, who published and did such a wonderful job on the orig-

inal manuscript of my first book, that's fine with me, but I know I did the work and put into action my creative talents. Then success was a combination; part me and part them. See what I mean?

Let's go a step further. If you are going to sit on your duff, waiting for someone to get you going, I think you'll wait a long time. I tell all of my students, "Bust your tail. Work hard every day of your life. Don't believe in fantasy, don't believe in fairy tales. Be real. Stick to your guns and give it all you've got. You'll be surprised at the results and you'll love the results." I know. I love my results.

WHO YOU KNOW IS NICE, WHAT YOU KNOW IS THE BEST, so if and when you make it, it will be the GREATEST SATISFACTION IN YOUR LIFE. That's what I believe.

Do You Get Embarrassed?

In all the eighty-two years of my life, I can't remember ever getting embarrassed. I have never experienced this form of emotion. I really do not know if it is one of our emotions, but whatever it may be I never find myself feeling embarrassed. Maybe I am too dumb to know why I should feel that way or recognize what would embarrass me. I honestly say I never have been in a position to feel that way.

I never knew what there was to get embarrassed about. I have never felt nervous, I have never felt "stage fright." So I can tell you, Sam Ulano never got embarrassed about anything he's done.

Why should I get embarrassed? I don't see any reason why. I do my thing to the best of my abilities and hope it comes out the best it can. That's all I can do. Nothing can make me feel unsure of myself. Nothing can break through my thick skull. I tell myself that I know my craft and so I am ready at all times. If I "fluff" on a lyric or "goof" at my drums, so what? I know I can do my thing and no one can embarrass me. NO WAY. NO HOW.

Does this sound strange to you? Do you think I'm making this up? SOLOMON P. ULANO aka SAM ULANO NEVER GETS EMBARRASSED. There's just no reason he should. I don't see any reason any of us should feel that way. No one will arrest us for doing something that we might get embarrassed about. I know no one will kill me and no one will chase me out of the room and no one will have me condemned. Of course, I do know that there are many of us who get embarrassed at things we do. We can't control ourselves because this is how we feel. However, we should investigate why we let this happen to us.

Just what is it that makes us cringe when we are embarrassed? It's interesting, because while some of us never, ever know that feeling, those who do get embarrassed never seem to know why this feeling comes through.

There is something in our makeup that happens — I don't know what or why — but it does take place. I've heard people say, "I NEVER WAS SO EMBARRASSED IN MY LIFE. I COULD DIE. IF THERE WAS A HOLE BIG ENOUGH I WOULD HAVE JUMPED IN IT. OH MY GOD, I WAS SO EMBARRASSED." So it goes. Not me. I am happy I don't feel this way. That's my PHILOSOPHY OF LIFE.

Do You Pray?

Interesting thought. DO YOU PRAY? If you are a believer in a Supreme Being, called GOD or whomever you think it is, I ask you, do you PRAY? "OH GOD. PLEASE HELP ME. I NEED YOUR HELP!" Whatever you say when and if you do pray. I know I pray and I know I believe very much that there is someone or something watching over me. I feel we all, in our privacy, pray and look up to heaven. "GOD, WHEREVER YOU ARE, PLEASE WATCH OVER ME."

I don't know about you out there, but every time I fly in the sky I pray that the LORD watches over me. I pray in my mind as the plane is taking off. I sort of hold on tightly to my seat and make sure my seat belt is tight and holding me in a secure position. Yes, I do pray and have prayed every day of my growing life. I remember when I was in the ARMY and heading overseas to unknown areas of the world. I really prayed pretty heavy then.

I wasn't alone. Almost all of the guys on the ship were very religious. We prayed all day. Many prayed in their beds as we were falling asleep. The war in the Pacific was heating up. We were in the 98th DIVISION, an Army combat division on a troop transport heading to invade JAPAN. Whether Catholic, Jew, or Muslim, everybody prayed, each to their GOD. We each were very, very serious and showed we all loved GOD and asked for help from the LORD.

I think it is very common that we pray to GOD. The person who tells me that they don't pray makes me think they are lying. Praying is healthy for our minds. It is healthy for our inner selves. We are very human when we pray. It's a real part of living.

There is nothing wrong or silly about praying. GOD is near to all of us. GOD makes us feel great and beautiful. That's what I believe. I really think GOD has guided me all the eighty-two years of my life. I know I wrote about this feeling and have always professed to my students, my family, and my loved ones, that I believe someone or something has been inside me all my life.

How can I account for all of this writing that I do? What makes me think as I do? I don't have the answers, but I feel that something inside my brain and body makes me believe this way. "Create, Sam," something says to me. "DO YOUR THING, SAM," MY INNER SELF TELLS ME. It is so real I can't give you any other reason for what I do and how I do it. My hands hit the typewriter and I look up and I've finished another page. GO EXPLAIN IT.

At eighty-two, going on eighty-three, my life is great, fun, and happy and I PRAY EVERY CHANCE I GET. YES, SAM ULANO DOES PRAY. And loves it.

You Have a Brain, Use It!

When I was a youngster, my family would always say to me, "YOU HAVE A BRAIN, USE IT." I never did use it and I never could use it. I never did much thinking. It never registered with me that my brain had the capacity to do what I now can do with it.

It just sat on top of my head. I never really made use of this wonderful part of our physical makeup. Then again, I never knew to what extent I could do things through my brain. However, as I got older and started to teach every day, I was learning how to experiment with my mind. I found out that I, like everyone else, had the capacity to wake up this sleeping machine.

I was amazed at what I could create. "Fantastic," I would say. SAM ULANO was able to create drum study work that made sense. I began to find new ways to say things, new ways to write study work for my instrument. This wonderful brain opened new doors for me and the next thing you knew, I was writing and enjoying my musical life. Many people thought I was completely MESHUGGE, (NUTS, IN YIDDISH). I know I wasn't insane and I knew I had the capabilities to develop many new concepts for my drum studies. Just great and great fun.

Every one of us has a brain and every one of us needs to wake up and make use of it. Some of us never get to the point where we put the switch on that makes the brain operate. Every so often the brain comes alive and every so often some of us see what's possible when the switch of the brain gets turned on.

No one will turn it on for you. Only you can make full use of your brain. I've seen what can happen when I get my brain going. It's just so exciting. "LOOK MOM, I'M THINKING . . . CREATING, USING MY MIND."

All of us have the same opportunity to develop our own thinking process; how we see things and what we think is very important in our lives. All we have to do is be honest with ourselves. Be real and sit down and use your brain. Who knows what heights you might reach? Do it and see what happens.

Keep Reminding Yourself That You Must Stay on Track

I don't know about you, but I always have conversations with myself. I don't let anyone know that I talk to myself because then they would really think I'm off my rocker. However, I have some of the most interesting talk sessions with myself.

One topic MYSELF and I discuss is that I must always remember never to get depressed. I tell myself that I have put so much of my life into what I love to do that I never want to let it get away from me. Then I tell myself, never forget your system of living, never overeat, don't go back to being three hundred twenty pounds again. I make sure I remind myself to keep all my medical appointments at THE VETERAN'S HOSPITAL. I tell myself, "Don't forget, I AM A DIABETIC, LEVEL TWO." I MUST NEVER MISS MY MEDICATION. I take it seven days a week. My list of reminders goes on and on every day. I make this a part of my philosophy of life and I live by it.

You'll find it a great thing to do. I remind myself about all the important things in my life. I sit in the bathroom and ask myself questions, such as, "Did I take my medication?" "Did I pay my phone bill?" "What will I write about?" All kinds of things run through my brain. I check them off, mentally. "Do this," and "Do that, Sam." "Don't forget to go to the printers, go to the Post Office," and so forth.

Sometimes ideas come to me. This is when I write these thoughts down on paper. I always have pen and pad with me whether I'm on a bus or on a plane; wherever I am, I have a way to document things I need to remind myself about.

I have been talking to myself every day for a long time now and I've got it down to a "science." I call it my "stay on top of things" system. Got to do it. As I type, I recheck my thoughts and I type and talk to myself. It keeps my brain awake, keeps ideas running through my head. I check off what I have done today. That's how I use this concept of talking to myself. You should try it. It's a wonderful way to keep on guard and cover all bases.

If you try it, you eventually will work it into your everyday existence. On my days off I rest my brain and body. Oh yes, I do have days where I don't do anything and this is very important because the brain must have a rest period. I still do my body exercises and also run down a list of what I'm going to do, either the next day or the following days. However, I use this as part of my resting. I don't call that working.

If I Knew at Twenty
What I Know at Eighty

Interesting statement. Now that I am eighty-two, I have learned quite a bit. Had I known in my younger days what I now know, I might have accomplished so much. I might have been a better drummer, might have written quite a few more books. I "could have been a contender," as was said in a famous movie. Most of us have no idea what heights we might reach in life. So if we thought we were very smart when we were young, it's not until we grow older that we realize how dumb we really were.

At eighty-two, I can write about life from this viewpoint. I don't say every one of us gets ". . . too soon old and too late smart," as the Dutch say. But what silly people we were in our young years!

Of course we couldn't be as smart at twenty as we become at eighty, because we have to live life before we can know something. When we're young, we think we know a lot, but man, we don't even know how to blow our noses. We are so immature we still have to depend on Mom and Pop until we get through those years of school, high school, college, and get our feet wet in the work world. We experiment with jobs, floundering from one job to the next.

Then we learn about love, sex, and our bodies. We go through some of the illnesses of growing up. Then our own family and kids go through the same thing we did. Interesting cycle. Those growing pains, man, it's really incredible how it all goes around in a circle.

What makes us different than our parents? In the game of life, some of us win and some of us lose. None of us are such great brains that we know what to expect of our future.

It would be so wonderful if we knew at twenty what we eventually learn when we are eighty. It takes time and it all comes down to taking care of the body and staying in top physical shape. To me that is the key to all of this. It's so easy to see that taking care of our health is a major step in helping us reach some sense of knowing what we want and can do with our lives.

So I say to you who are reading this, you too must discover what life is all about. Maybe you'll learn it faster than I did. It could happen, you know. Above all, USE WHAT YOU LEARN.

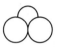

Have a Second Typewriter As a Backup, Just in Case

Here is something I realized was very important. I own a BROTHER 79 TYPEWRITER and have made such good use of it. However, about a month or so ago, my BROTHER 79 seemed to be showing signs of every so often not performing as well as I would have liked. I got a second, backup BROTHER 79 TYPEWRITER just in case I needed to write and ran into some problems with the first one. Now I always have a machine that works. The first one is still working well, but as they say, you never know. So that's the reason for the backup system.

I'm a big believer in having something that allows me to continue my work. Having the extra unit is so great because it allows me to keep going without interruption. It's a good idea that you all may put to use. I always say: "Two dollars are better than only one." We can all agree on this. When I get a chance I will get a third unit and this way I'll have a backup for the backup!

I say what the BOY SCOUTS and THE MARINES say, "ALWAYS READY." It can't hurt. It's like chicken soup, IT COULDN'T HOIT.

That feeling that things can run smoothly for you describes my concept of having the backup ready all the time. Knowing that you have the machines, ribbons for fast changing (literally in seconds), makes this a wonderful setup.

You say you do not think you'll ever do something like what I am doing? Well, I never thought I would write Book One or Book Two. I never ever gave it a thought. So you see, it can happen to you.

One of my dear friends said that when he got my first book, he was inspired and said he was going to get started on his life in music, with thousands of photographs. He said my book inspired him to get his book together and start to organize it and write the captions for the pictures. I told him that was a great idea and now we shall see when and what he puts together. I am certain it will be a work of art and an important document about the music scene over many years. **"GO FOR IT, MY MAN."**

Are You Jealous of Others?

I think I have been a very lucky man because I never have been jealous of others. I feel so fortunate that this was never one of the negative parts of my life. I don't think I could be jealous of others because it would make me very unhappy.

I can understand it, though, when people feel this way, but I feel that jealousy can make a person feel very disgruntled. Living my life that way would destroy my belief in myself and my belief that sometimes in my life I'll get a chance to prove myself. Instead, I let my mind be free of thinking that others got their chance ahead of me.

More power to everyone who does what I do. They should all get accolades for their abilities. This is how I have felt all of my life. Being jealous of other people, as I see it, is having our brain and mental attitudes diverted from TAKING CARE OF OUR OWN ABILITIES AND TALENTS.

Furthermore, I think it's dangerous if we spend a significant part of our lives being jealous of someone else. Even if I felt someone wasn't as deserving as I am and that person got what I wanted, I still wouldn't feel jealous. The reason I think jealousy is not healthy for us is that our mind, brain, and gut can't and shouldn't have to handle this feeling. I see people getting sick when their nervous system and emotions get all twisted.

Talk to your doctors and see what they think about this problem. Maybe they can give you advice on how to undo this terrible feeling.

Being jealous doesn't help anyone's situation. In fact, it can destroy a person's enjoyment of what they do. I like to keep free of these harmful ideas. Sometimes when we feel this way we bad-mouth our fellow workers. We say things that later on we regret. Not a good thing.

How Do You See Yourself?

I was once asked how I see myself. At first I felt a little strange in answering this question, but after a while I did have an answer. I always THOUGHT I saw myself as someone who studied hard and someone who knows what I am about.

In my thirties I started to understand myself. I began to know what the strong points in my life were. I knew that if I practiced hard and studied, I stood a good chance of reaching some of my early goals.

My philosophy of life started to take better shape as I reached fifty and sixty years of age. I still didn't think I had all the pieces of the puzzle in place at that time, but I did feel that I was finding out more about myself. Little by little, this showed up in my daily life. Of course now, at eighty-two, I understand a lot better what I am about and where I am heading.

I think once we know who we are we can accomplish many things. Of course, if we are not honest with ourselves, we sometimes never find ourselves and go on searching for years.

How do I see myself? I see myself as a person who can use his abilities in the music field at a high professional level. I get up every day and retrace the steps of the days before. I have learned that review is one of the secrets of a better life. **Over and over, again and again.** Sounds like you read this somewhere in my first book? I can't help myself, because I know now that this is the secret for **Sam Ulano.**

Somewhere in the Bible it says, **"Know Thyself."** Knowing ourselves tells us that we might be able to reach heights we never thought we could reach. It's important that we know everything about ourselves. Why we get angry, why we never finish what we start, why we can do the things we can do, and why we can't do some other things. Find out what your strong points and your faults are. Find out how to correct what needs correcting. Don't think anyone on this earth hasn't any faults. **WE ALL HAVE THEM.** Man, do we have faults.

Sy Oliver, the famous band leader and arranger said: **"IT'S SO EASY WHEN WE KNOW HOW."** This is so true. I now know myself very well and I have no problem facing every day. **NO PROBLEM AT ALL.**

"Simplicity," Dizzy Gillespie Said to One of His Drummers

Some time ago, at the original BIRDLAND, on 7th Avenue and 52nd Street, here in New York City, DIZZY GILLESPIE was working with his band. The drummer, not too experienced, but a great talent, sort of over-played the band arrangement and in a certain spot, this drummer tried to do some complicated involved drum solo to boost up the beat. His stick went flying out of his hand and all hell broke loose. The band finished the set and were leaving the bandstand when DIZZY yelled at the drummer, "SIMPLICITY, MON. Don't try to play the entire arrangement in one or two measures."

It was fun listening to DIZZY tell the young player to take it easy and not to try to do too much in a short passage of music. I was standing near this young fellow as he came off the stage and he said to me, "DIZZY IS SO RIGHT."

There was a good lesson to be learned not only for the drummer who goofed up but for myself and a few of us who were listening to the maestro, DIZZY, when he asked his players to KEEP IT SIMPLE, MON. EASY DOES IT. DON'T TRY TO EAT THE ENTIRE STEAK IN ONE BITE. It makes sense to me because it is easier to ride on the sound of the band. Of course this is not only in music. It fits into all fields of endeavor. Try to keep things easy, flexible, and not overdone. Nice and simple. Don't over-complicate the situation and you can't go wrong.

I understand this simplicity business. It is the surest method to staying on top.

DIZZY SAID IT SO NICELY. He didn't get angry at the young drum player. He told him like it was. If you are going to reach for the stars, you must make sure you can do it. Reach, but keep it simple and musical when in a musical situation. Let yourself have some space. Don't crowd yourself. Do what is within your abilities. Have the mental sense to "cool it" and keep it simple, as DIZZY said. It works better and gives you the opportunity to try and make the simplest things fit the tune.

Allow yourself the simple feel, play musically, and don't over-complicate things. The more you stay within your capabilities, the better things work out. Then, there's less chance for slipups and less chance to screw things up.

I like this idea because I can do my thing and make it sound so wonderful. "GIVE ME THE SIMPLE LIFE," as the song says. The great performers in music, in art, in business, in all areas of life know this is true.

Start at the Age of Fifteen or Sixteen

I have done a great deal of talking about staying in physical shape using light free weights, such as ten pounds, fifteen pounds, and twenty pounds. Someone asked me at what age I thought someone should start a program of light free weights. That's a good question and I should address it at this time. Let me back up a bit.

People under fourteen years of age shouldn't do too much weight lifting. Of course you must realize that this is my opinion and concept of how I think this development should be handled. Young people don't have the stamina just yet, and I feel it is important that any of this body work should first be directed by a coach who knows how to explain how this should be done.

Before you think of even getting into this idea of body training, I advise one and all to check with your doctor. It's important that you are checked and told you are in condition to handle this training program. Don't just go into it without seeing your doctor. For myself, I have myself checked three or four times a year. The doctors check my heart, blood pressure, eyes, ears, my whole body. I need a clear approval that it's okay for me to go on with my body training.

Okay, so we have the doctor tell us it's all right for us to train. Now if you are just starting out, a ten minute, or tops, fifteen minute routine is sufficient. I'd advise **NO MORE FOR AT LEAST TWO OR THREE MONTHS.**

I tell my students that after the age of fifteen or sixteen, you are in the age range to get into free weights. A slow but simple system is what you want in the beginning and no more. I do it every day, a steady ten-minute program. I lift the ten-pound weights ten times and then I stop. I lift the fifteen-pound weights again for ten reps (REPS mean repetitions). I suggest ten lifts with the

217

twenty pounds and then stop. So what I'm telling you after the age of fifteen or sixteen, it is good to get into FREE WEIGHTS . . . WITH MODERATION. That means, no hard workouts.

Some of you might do some running after lifting the weights. Running is good aerobics. I've stopped my running program. At eighty-two, going on eighty-three, I find the running routine a bit dangerous for me. I also think it's not too good for most seniors. I've stayed with the light free weights. I've found it's good for my legs and my whole body. You too will find this is the best way to stay in shape.

Read the physical fitness magazines sold on newsstands. They give you some interesting ideas about staying in condition. You will gain from this if you set up a program. But remember, if you are under the age of fifteen or sixteen, lifting weights is not the best idea.

The Amazing Brain

Throughout my writing about my philosophy of life, I have constantly made reference to THE BRAIN. I call it the HUMAN COMPUTER. The BRAIN directs us in how we think, what we want to do, how to create, and how to use our imagination. Our brain is so great because it can do things that no other part of our bodies can do. It can help us learn anything we want to learn.

The computer we buy in a store keeps getting better and better. IT'S FANTASTIC, BUT IT'S IMPORTANT TO KNOW THAT THE COMPUTER WE BUY CAN ONLY DO SOMETHING IF WE PLUG IT INTO A SOCKET.

Now look at the brain. We can take our brain with us no matter where we want to go. Our brain doesn't need a wire to plug it into a socket. We can lie in bed and our brain is on. It doesn't shut down, sometimes even when we are asleep. It's wonderful.

In fact, the computer we buy in a store is limited only to what the human brain wishes to insert into the machine. Most of us realize that the computer can only do limited things.

The human brain can do what we want, any time, any place, any hour of the day or night. Its possibilities are endless. Think about this: Our brain can correct our mistakes, in writing, in speaking, in thinking, or whatever needs correcting, as many times as corrections have to be made.

Yes, I know the many things that a computer can do, but all of those things must first be programmed ahead of time. While the computer has limitations, the brain can do the things a computer cannot do. It's marvelous.

More About the Brain

I have some very interesting thoughts about our brain. For example: We can have a heart transplant and go on living; we can get a new liver, kidney; even sew an arm back on. Many parts of the body can be replaced but we can't replace the brain. In a computer we can get rid of the computer we have and buy the latest model, but we can't buy a new brain. Fascinating, isn't it? We have the brain we are born with and that's all we have. There are no second chances for purchasing a new one.

When we are born, we are told that we must develop the one brain we have. We either do that or nothing is going to develop for us. We might stay stupid or we might become the world's greatest "brain." Then again, we may just be like most everyone else, just average.

Each year after my thirteenth birthday, I began to find myself more and more. I found out that I wasn't as dumb as I thought I was. I could think and I could learn whatever I wanted to learn. As the years passed I came to the conclusion that my brain could think up ideas about playing my instrument. In fact, I found I was thinking so far ahead of my fellow drum players that now they really thought I was nuts!

Interestingly, before I was thirteen years old, I and everybody else, my family, school teachers, and friends that I grew up with, all felt that I was never going to amount to anything in my life. Of course, I fooled all of them. This brain I was born with woke up. It started to come alive. There were ideas brewing in this brain of mine.

I started to write and create my early books about playing drums. I didn't read much literature about olden drums. I wasn't very interested in what took place with drums thousands of years ago. I was living in the present. I was years ahead of my fellow percussionists. The way I knew this, most of the better players looked upon me as a freak on drums. I could play quite well, but where I differed from the other players was that I was experimenting with new approaches to studying and getting better.

This is when I recognized that the BRAIN I HAD WAS VERY ADVANCED. I just had to learn how to use it. Thus all my ideas began percolating and bubbling in the kettle over my shoulders. So now I realized that my BRAIN COMPUTER, THE LIVE AND ACTIVE COMPUTER, WAS DOING SOMETHING FOR ME. What was great was that I didn't have to buy an up-to-date computer. I didn't need any MICROSOFT PARTS. None of that stuff. My brain computer updated itself.

Man! This was starting to be fun for me.

Even More About the Brain

A human brain is required to activate a computer. The wires must be plugged into a socket and then a human person must throw the switch. Now we have the computer working. Our brain doesn't need any wires or switches. OUR BRAIN IS ALWAYS ON. All of us just have to understand the possibilities of the human brain.

I am so excited about my future, and I wait in wonderment to see what my human brain will be thinking of five or ten years from now. Who knows? I might do Book Five about my philosophy in the next few years. You never can tell. The future of my life is so marvelous as far as I can see it. I know I'm not clairvoyant, and I know I can't possibly predict the future, but my human brain may be able to steer me into new, uncharted waters of life.

Since I have been able to do what I have done thus far, I can never tell what I might conceive of in the next five or ten years of my life. A lot depends on the condition of my brain. It also depends on what condition my body will be in at that time. As far as that is concerned, I intend to make every effort to stay on top of my physical fitness program. I will not get drunk, and I do not plan to go back to smoking. I will keep my body program going at full speed ahead.

So putting all of this together, I think my future looks very bright. I don't know about you guys and gals reading this, but for me, I see it being a very rosy future, and I feel I'll be very successful at reaching my goals. Who's to say I can't achieve these goals? Only I can be the judge.

Let's look at what is in store for those of us who start to understand our brain and thought capabilities. No one can say we haven't the talent to discover what we are trying to discover.

Is there an answer to all of this? I say, yes! THINK WITH YOUR BRAIN. USE YOUR IMAGINATION. DEVELOP YOUR CREATIVE SKILLS. TRY TO UNDERSTAND WHAT YOU ARE ABOUT. DISCOVER AND UNCOVER GREAT THOUGHTS ABOUT THE FIELD YOU ARE IN.

The main thing about all of this is to know you have the great brain that should and can be utilized. Once you realize all of this you are on your way. Take it from me, YOUR BRAIN WILL BE YOUR KEY and ideas will do the trick — for you and for me.

Sam Ulano

Taking up the drums at age 13, SAM ULANO opened his first studio four years later and began teaching and writing about drumming. He followed up high school with four years at the Manhattan School of Music before being drafted into the army, where he trained a 100-piece drum corps.

Now 84 years old and showing no signs of letting up, Sam is a performer, educator and author who has been in the music profession for over 65 years. During that time, he has studied with and taught the best of them, while carving out a niche for himself as a respected drummer on the New York scene. Sam has played at many of the top nightspots in New York, including the Gaslight Club and, currently, the famed Red Blazer. He's played the summer resorts, the concert field, and is known as "Mr. Rhythm" for his more than 500 shows for young audiences throughout the New York school system. He has appeared on television with Steve Allen on *The Tonight Show*, as well as with Gary Moore, Ernie Kovacs, and Joe Franklin.

Well-known for his methods of drum teaching and his progressive approach to writing about the instrument he loves, Sam has over 2500 instruction books to his credit — 300 in the past five years alone! He also has produced records, audio and video tapes, and CDs of his instruction and performance. He continues to write, teach, and perform in his own inimitable style.

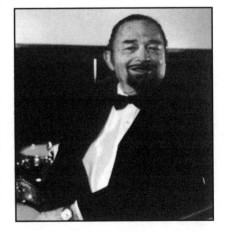

Letters From
Friends and Family

Your book comforted me — simple, yet the words felt warm. You have a way of making everyday life . . . manifest good.

– Fern Tishma

My brother Sam has done it again. But this time, my wife Anita and I think this book is better than his first book. Book one is more closely related to the technical part and book two relates to a person's approach to life. This book is inspirational. Keep up writing Sam. Best of luck.

– Ben Ulano

I think your book contains a lot of things that people can use to help with their lives. The problem with most people is that they don't have the motivation and discipline to carry out a program for an extended period of time.

Your life experience – how you have followed up on your career and worked all the time to improve your ability in the drumming field – should help motivate your readers. The fact that at your age you still can perform well should make most people feel they can follow your philosophies and do the same.

Keep going. We are always interested in what you are doing and happy with your success.

– Sol Ulano

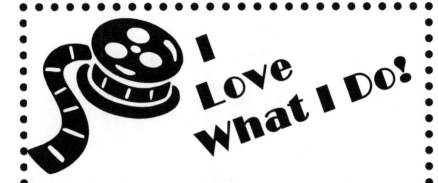

Premieres Fall 2005

A feature length documentary film, I LOVE WHAT I DO!, focusing on Sam and his life in the world of music, is currently in post production and is scheduled for completion in Fall of 2005.

Produced and Directed by Sam's Academy Award winning son, Mark Ulano, the film is a musical meditation on mentorship, happiness, the arts and their impact on family life.

The video will be available for purchase on
www.samulano.com
immediately upon release.

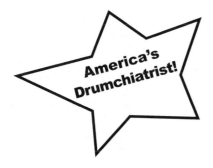

America's Drumchiatrist!

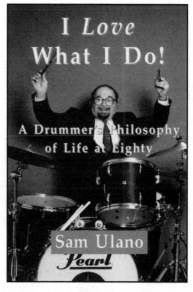

I Love
What I Do!

A Drummer's Philosophy
of Life at Eighty

Sam Ulano

I Love What I Do!
A Drummer's Philosophy
Of Life at Eighty
Sam Ulano
168 pgs, 1-890995-35-5
$14.95

America loves Sam, the *Drumchiatrist,* and his inspiring philosophy! This is a book about living life with joy and enthusiasm. Long revered both personally and professionally as a teacher and drummer extraordinaire, Sam has taken his lifetime of experiences and drum rolled them into this exuberant book of practical suggestions for getting more out of life – for staying healthier, for learning new skills, for making a living, for having more fun! Vital and productive at 80, Sam is his own best advertisement, and in his optimistic, friendly and honest way he isn't shy about "telling it like it is," while reminding us of the wonderful world in which we live.

For Sam Ulano's books, manuals and recordings, visit:
www.samulano.com

If You Enjoyed *Keep Swinging*, Check Out These Great Titles!

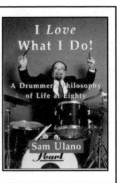
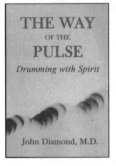
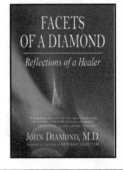
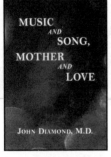